Studies in Maritime Literary History,

1760-1930

© Acadiensis Press 1991

Canadian Cataloguing in Publication Data

Main entry under title:

Studies in Maritime literary history

      Includes bibliographical references.
      ISBN 0-919107-34-6

1. Canadian literature (English) — Maritime
Provinces — History and criticism. * I. Davies,
Gwendolyn.

PS8131.M3S78 1991   C810.9'9715   C91-097630-9
PR9198.2.M3S78 1991

Cover design:
Julie Scriver

Studies in Maritime Literary History,

1760-1930

Gwendolyn Davies

Acadiensis Press
Fredericton, New Brunswick
1991

for

Cyril Davies

and

Wilhelmina Babbitt (Nordin) Davies

ACKNOWLEDGEMENTS

Over the years, there are many people whom one wants to thank for assistance and support. The Bell and Crake Funds at Mount Allison University, the AUFA Research Fund at Acadia University, and the SSHRC/Small Universities Grant at Acadia University have made it possible for me to conduct research and to participate in conference proceedings. A SSHRC Leave Fellowship in my sabbatical year, 1984-85, made it possible for me to do the work on satirists that eventually resulted in publications on Thomas McCulloch, the Club group, and James Irving.

The combined Library and Archives staffs of many institutions, particularly those of Mount Allison University, Acadia University, the Public Archives of Nova Scotia, and Dalhousie University have provided invaluable assistance. In particular, I want to thank Margaret Fancy, Special Collections, and Cheryl Ennals, Archives, at Mount Allison; Allan Dunlop, Archivist, at the Public Archives of Nova Scotia; and Pat Townsend, University Archivist, and Edith Haliburton, Special Collections, at Acadia for their constant interest and support. Beryl MacFadden, English Department Secretary at Mount Allison, typed a number of these articles for me between 1976 and 1988. Since then, and particularly in the preparation of this book, I owe Joy Cavazzi, Secretary of the Department of English at Acadia, an enormous debt of gratitude for her patience and her efforts in typing papers for presentation or publication. I also want to express my appreciation to Dr. Phillip Buckner, Acadiensis Press, for his guidance and support throughout the collation of material for this selection of essays. Clara Thomas, my thesis supervisor at York University, has always been an inspiration.

Finally, I wish to express my warmest thanks to Dr. Margaret Conrad, Department of History, Acadia University, and to Michael J. Hellyer, Academic Relations Officer, Canadian High Commission, London, without whose encouragement this book would not have been produced.

Gwendolyn Davies
Acadia University
December 1991

PERMISSIONS

I wish to thank the following for permission to reprint essays:

"Persona in Planter Journals," from Margaret Conrad, ed., *They Planted Well* (Fredericton: Acadiensis Press, 1988).

"Consolation to Distress: Loyalist Literary Activity in the Maritimes," from *Acadiensis*, Vol. XVI, No. 2 (Spring 1987).

"'Dearer Than His Dog': Literary Women in Pre-Confederation Nova Scotia," from Barbara Godard, ed., *Gynocritics/ La Gynocritique* (Toronto: ECW Press, 1987).

"James Irving: Literature and Libel in Early Nova Scotia," from *Essays on Canadian Writing*, No. 29 (Summer 1984).

"The Club Papers: Haliburton's Literary Apprenticeship," from Frank M. Tierney, ed., *The Thomas Chandler Haliburton Symposium* (Ottawa: University of Ottawa Press, 1985).

"William Charles M'Kinnon: Cape Breton's Sir Walter Scott," from *Collections of the Royal Nova Scotia Historical Society*, Vol. 41 (1982).

"The Dodge Club and the Tradition of Nineteenth-Century American Travel Literature," Introduction to James DeMille, *The Dodge Club or Italy in MDCCCLIX* (Sackville: R.P. Bell Library, Mount Allison University, 1981).

"'A Past Of Orchards': Rural Change in Maritime Literature before Confederation," from Peter Thomas, ed., *The Red Jeep and Other Landscapes: A Collection in Honour of Douglas Lochhead* (Sackville and Fredericton: The Centre for Canadian Studies, Mount Allison University, and Goose Lane Editions Ltd., 1987).

"The Song Fishermen: A Regional Poetry Celebration," from Larry McCann, ed., *People and Place: Studies of Small Town Life in the Maritimes* (Fredericton: Acadiensis Press, 1987).

"Afterword: *Rockbound*," from Frank Parker Day, *Rockbound* (Toronto: University of Toronto Press, 1989).

Table of Contents

Introduction:
Steering to Our Sources

On New Year's Day in 1848, Nova Scotian whaler Benjamin Doane and his fellow crewmen went to the racetrack in Sydney, Australia, and found one of the favourites there named "Sam Slick." "So to the Antipodes —," notes Doane, "whether round the Horn or by the Cape of Good Hope, or both — had the fame of the great 'Bluenose' writer, Judge Haliburton, borne the name of his homely hero."[1] Six years later, Doane's Barrington, Nova Scotia, townsman, Jacob Norton Crowell, attended an auction on the goldfields of Ballarat, Australia, and found amongst the items for sale several copies of Haliburton's "Sam Slick" costing 4s.6d. each.[2] That two men from the same small coastal community in Nova Scotia should encounter the handiwork of their literary countryman half way around the world demonstrates not only the mobility that has always informed the lifestyle of Canada's Maritime Provinces but also the degree to which a nineteenth-century Maritime writer could, within a few years of publication, become known beyond regional borders. While one cannot ignore the publishing limitations facing a number of authors on the east coast of Canada in the nineteenth century, there nonetheless exists in the universal popularity of Haliburton's Sam Slick sketches, the British recognition of Moses Perley's New Brunswick sporting sketches,[3] the international popularity of Lucy Maud Montgomery's *Anne of Green Gables*,[4] and the transatlantic publication of such nineteenth and early twentieth century writers as Marshall Saunders, Alice Jones, James DeMille, Bliss Carman, and Charles G.D. Roberts, evidence of the profile that many pre-1930s Maritime writers achieved in the literary field.

This selection of essays emerges from fifteen years of archival, periodical, and textual research into the wealth of imaginative material that English-speaking Maritimers read, wrote, and savoured in the period from 1760 to 1930. The dates of the selection are invariably arbitrary, reflecting for the early period an interest in the eight thousand New England Planters who took up the lands of the deported Acadians after 1759-60, and culminating in the

---

1   Benjamin Doane, *Following the Sea* (Halifax, 1987), p. 162.

2   Jacob Norton Crowell, "Pencillings on Sea and Shore, or a Voyage to Australia (Journal of a Digger)," Evelyn Richardson Papers, MG 1, Vol. 1419, ts., p. 83, PANS.

3   John William Carleton, ed. *The Sporting Sketch Book: A Series of Characteristic Papers* (London, 1842), p. iii-iv. In his "Preface," Carleton says that he approached for inclusion in his book "one of the most graceful and imaginative writers that ever touched and embellished sporting subjects." He adds in a note: "Need I say I speak of Mr. M.H. Perley, the 'New Brunswicker'?"

4   See: Yuko Katsura, "Red-haired Anne in Japan," *Canadian Children's Literature*, 34 (1984), pp. 57-60; and, "L.M. Montgomery: at home in Poland," *Canadian Children's Literature*, 46 (1987), pp. 7-36.

shifting literary responses to the region following the labour unrest, financial stringency, and outmigration of the 1920s. The essays therefore mark personal stages in literary discovery. Inevitably, they reflect gaps in the periods and range of material covered. For instance, neither the post-Confederation Fredericton poets nor the late nineteenth-century "New Women" writers are covered in the essays in this selection, although glancing reference to both will be made in the introduction.

In writing about Maritime literature, one is inevitably faced with the question: Is there a distinctive Maritime culture? For the average Maritimer, this is probably not a significant question. Being a Maritimer is a matter of knowing, of being. It is something "bred in the bone," or as writers Charles Bruce and Alistair MacLeod variously put it, it is the "salt in the blood" or the "salt gift of blood."[5] Implicit in these words is a sense of rootedness, of geographical and historical belonging. "There is nothing superficial about a Maritimer's common and deep sense of place," noted former Trent professor Alan Wilson in 1982, "his sensitivity to family and local tradition, his sense of bond with New England and of suspicion of Upper Canada, and his wariness toward governments, even his own."[6] Warning in both his poetry and prose that "Words are never enough" to capture what he calls "The essence of Maritime Canada," writer Charles Bruce nonetheless notes in "Atlantic Cadence": "If there is one thing known in common it must be the sound of water, the beaches, from Bay Chaleur down the coasts of New Brunswick and the Island, round the headlands of Cape North, down the eastern and southern shores and round the coast of Fundy to Passamaquoddy and the edge of Maine. The grumbling sigh of calm bays at night, the rush of millbrooks and the soft slap on the shores of lakes. The sound of rivers that run to the beat of their names, Matapedia and Kennebecasis, Medway and Margaree."[7]

Having said as much, Bruce goes on to warn against generalization. To some, the Maritimes are "the feel of a scythe in timothy." To others, they are "the creek and thump of rowlocks in fog." Steel, coal, and industry have been added to "a land-sea economy of intense diversity," resulting in a quality of adaptability that Bruce sees as central to the Maritime inheritance.[8] Or as Haliburton put it in *The Old Judge* in 1849, "The Nova Scotian...is often found superintending the cultivation of a farm and building a vessel at the

---

5   See: Charles Bruce, *The Mulgrave Road* (Porter's Lake, Nova Scotia, 1985), pp. 50-52; and Alistair MacLeod, *The Lost Salt Gift of Blood* (Toronto, 1976).

6   Alan Wilson, "Cross Currents in Maritime Regionalism" quoted in William B. Hamilton, *Regional Identity: A Maritime Quest* (Sackville, New Brunswick, 1985), p. 10.

7   Charles Bruce, "Atlantic Cadence," Charles Bruce Papers, Dal. MS 2, 297, E.20, Dalhousie University Archives.

8   *Ibid.*

same time; and is not only able to catch and cure a cargo of fish, but to find his way with it to the West Indies or the Mediterranean; he is a man of all work, but expert in none — knows a little of many things, but nothing well."[9] But above all, Bruce argues, there is inheritance — a sense of continuity with family, place, or tradition that survives both outmigration and the cosmopolitan flair of the returnees, existing "somewhere deep in the soundless well of knowing."[10] "We are our pasts," adds poet George Elliott Clarke, in 1990, "Nothing is forgotten."[11]

As the essay on the "home place" in this selection will argue, a sense of this past, this rootedness, is one of the things to emerge from a reading of modern as well as early Maritime literature. Imbued with a consciousness of who they were and where they were, Maritime writers from the eighteenth century onward began to define themselves in relation to the region. Most in this period were newcomers to the country who brought with them as part of their intellectual baggage the literary forms and cultural expectations of their British, American or other backgrounds. Thus, one may find a tension between anticipation and realization in poems such as Joseph Stansbury's "To Cordelia" (1780s)[12] or the Bard MacLean's "The Gloomy Forest" (c. 1819-48),[13] for "Plenty" did not always sit "Queen/O'er as happy a country as ever was seen," as *The Gentleman's Magazine* of February 1750 promised.[14] On the whole, however, these disillusionments were the exception rather than the rule in early Maritime writing, and the majority of people, whatever their backgrounds, were busily engaged in getting on with life in the new world. Maritime literature of the early period reflects these social and domestic preoccupations, typically illustrating in the Saint John marriage poem of Anne Hecht (1786), the Saint John theatre prologue of Anonymous (1795), the Annapolis Royal tribute of Roger Viets (1788), or the Hudibrastic satire on New Lights of Jacob Bailey (c. 1784), a range of writing directed at the manners and mores of society.[15] In 1791, a tribute to Nova

---

9   Thomas Chandler Haliburton, *The Old Judge or Life in a Colony* (Ottawa, 1978), p. xxi.

10 Charles Bruce, *The Mulgrave Road*, p. 52.

11 George Elliott Clarke, *Whylah Falls* (Winlaw, British Columbia, 1990), p. 16.

12 Joseph Stansbury, "To Cordelia" in Winthrop Sargent, ed., *The Loyal Verses of Joseph Stansbury And Doctor Jonathan Odell* (Albany, 1860), p. 90-1.

13 "John MacLean's 'Gloomy Forest'," *The Dalhousie Review*, 28 (1948-49), pp. 158-162.

14 "Nova Scotia. A New Ballad," *The Gentleman's Magazine*, (February 1750), p. 84.

15 See: Anne Hecht, "Advice to Mrs. Mowat," in Grace Helen Mowat, *The Diverting History of a Loyalist Town* (Fredericton, 1953), pp. 56-58; Anonymous, "Prologue On Opening a Little Theatre In This City, on Monday The 5th January Inst." *The Royal Gazette and the New-Brunswick Advertiser*, IX, No. CCCCLV (20 January 1795), p. 4; Roger Viets, *Annapolis Royal* (Kingston, 1979) [1788]); Jacob Bailey, "Verse Against the New Lights" in George A. Rawlyk, *New Light Letters and Songs* (Hantsport, Nova Scotia, 1983), pp. 302-303.

Scotian poet, Pollio, provided an inadvertent glimpse of a Halifax polluted by hundreds of coal and wood-burning fires: "And hearest thou, Pollio, in the smoky town/Acadia's wild romantic sweets cry down?"[16] In 1804, Judge Alexander Croke's long poem, "The Inquisition," revealingly satirized the peccadillos of the Halifax elite, particularly the Governor's lady, Frances Wentworth;[17] and, in 1820, former Blackwood's litterateur, James Irving, brought to the Nova Scotian newspaper public his personal interpretations of Wordsworth, Coleridge, Shelley, and the Romantic revolution in English poetry.[18] In his "Conclusion" to the *Literary History of Canada*, Northrop Frye argues that "In the Canadas, even in the Maritimes, the frontier was all around one, a part and a condition of one's whole imaginative being."[19] In fact, in few Maritime works of the eighteenth or early nineteenth centuries is this sentiment illustrated. There is no Susanna Moodie in the Maritimes searching for reassuring evidence of "filagree," "privet," or "lignum-vitae" amongst the shrubbery, trying to accommodate herself to new experiences that numb her imagination.[20] There is no Catharine Parr Traill in Maritime literature penetrating the wilderness, insisting as she goes that "we have neither fay nor fairy, ghost nor bogle, satyr nor wood-nymph; our very forests disdain to shelter dryad or hama-dryad"[21] — and, thereby, in their absence, feeling compelled to fill the silence with her own words, her own mythologies.

Instead, in the Maritimes there was Thomas McCulloch's Mephibosheth Stepsure, a feisty persona who in Letter 23 had little patience with Parnassus and even less with dryads. Indeed, McCulloch's 1821 persona was fully preoccupied with his errant gadding-about neighbours, who in their drinking, gambling, frolicking, gossiping way failed to meet his self-imposed standards of economic and moral respectability. McCulloch's 25 letters published in the *Acadian Recorder* between 1821 and 1823 owed their success not only to the dry wit and tartness of their satire (the letters laid the foundation of Canadian humour, according to Northrop Frye),[22] but also to the sophistication of their

---

16 B., "Spring. A Nova-Scotia Pastoral," *The Nova-Scotia Magazine*, IV (July 1791), p. 441.

17 "Alexander Croke, *The Inquisition*" in Thomas B. Vincent, ed., *Narrative Verse Satire in Maritime Canada, 1779-1814* (Ottawa, 1978), pp. 143-172.

18 I—G, "Letters on the Present State of English Poetry," *The Acadian Recorder* (May 13, 1820 - October 19, 1822).

19 Northrop Frye, "Conclusion" in Carl F. Klinck, ed., *Literary History of Canada*, II (Toronto, 1976), p. 338.

20 Susanna Moodie, *Roughing It In The Bush* (Toronto, 1966 [1852]), p. 26.

21 Catharine Parr Traill, "Matter-Of-Fact Country" in Carl F. Klinck and Reginald E. Watters, eds., *Canadian Anthology* (Toronto, 1974), p. 26.

22 H. Northrop Frye, "Introduction" in Thomas McCulloch, *The Stepsure Letters* (Toronto, 1960), p. ix. This edition published only sixteen letters. The full 25 letters are available in

nineteenth-century Maritime reading audience, long schooled to responding to satirical newspaper sketches over its morning coffee. "We looked with great anxiety for the arrival of the 'Recorder'," noted one contemporary of McCulloch's, "and on its receipt used to assemble in the shop of Mr. — to hear 'Stepsure' read, and pick out the characters, and comment on their foibles, quite sure that they were among ourselves." "Great was often the anger expressed," he added, "and threats uttered against the author if they could discover him."[23]

In a sense, the Mephibosheth Stepsure letters mark a watershed in nineteenth-century Maritime literature, representing on one hand the climax of 40 years of post-Loyalist writing on the follies and foibles of society, while at the same time setting a new standard by which the narrative newspaper satires of the Club group (1828-31) and Thomas Chandler Haliburton (1835) would be measured. However, there is little sense of this development in Northrop Frye's "Conclusion" to the *Literary History of Canada* where Frye hypothesizes that "Canada has, for all practical purposes, no Atlantic seaboard. The traveller from Europe edges into it like a tiny Jonah entering an inconceivably large whale, slipping past the Straits of Belle Isle into the Gulf of St. Lawrence, where five Canadian provinces surround him, for the most part invisible.... To enter the United States is a matter of crossing an ocean; to enter Canada is a matter of being silently swallowed by an alien continent."[24]

Dramatic as Frye's image is, it fails to address the situation on the Atlantic seaboard. Whales do abound in the nineteenth-century sea journals of such writers as Benjamin Doane and Joshua Slocum,[25] but, elsewhere, neither whales, Jonahs, nor alien continents emerge as central to the iconography of early Maritime literature. As Janice Kulyk Keefer points out in *Under Eastern Eyes*, "anyone who reads much of the literature of this region becomes aware of how resistant the Maritime imagination is to such ideas as that of an alien continent dominated by a terrifying wilderness which for Frye forms the *sine qua non* of the Canadian imagination."[26] Indeed, when Emily Beavan of Long Creek published her 1845 *Life in the Backwoods of New Brunswick*, she wrote not of an alien environment but of pioneer efforts to move a house on log rollers, of the arrival by post of American newspapers and novel serializations, or of the presence in a settler's simple dwelling of a

Thomas McCulloch, *The Mephibosheth Stepsure Letters*, ed. Gwendolyn Davies (Ottawa, 1990).

23 William McCulloch, *Life of Thomas McCulloch, D.D., Pictou* (Truro, 1920), p. 73.

24 Northrop Frye, "Conclusion." p. 336.

25 Joshua Slocum, *Sailing Alone Around The World* (New York, 1956 [1900]), p. 150-51.

26 Janice Kulyk Keefer, *Under Eastern Eyes* (Toronto 1987), p. 27.

"Sam Slick, of Slickville...wooden-made yankee" clock.[27] Hers is not Susanna Moodie's garrison mentality, captured succinctly at the end of *Roughing It In The Bush* in the comment: "If these sketches should prove the means of deterring one family from sinking their property, and shipwrecking all their hopes, by going to reside in the backwoods of Canada I shall consider myself amply repaid for revealing the secrets of the prison-house, and feel that I have not toiled and suffered in the wilderness in vain."[28] Rather, in Beavan's work there is an expression of the same confidence in the future that took Oliver Goldsmith's "lonely settler" from his "wilderness of trees" in 1825 to the prosperity of "his wide barn with ample treasures filled" some 50 years later.[29] Haliburton makes it clear in the first pages of the *Old Judge*, notes Janice Kulyk Keefer, that "he is writing of civilized life in Nova Scotia."[30] Although pioneer conditions may still be found in the interior, remarks Haliburton, "yet the country has passed the period of youth and may now be called an old colony."[31]

No better illustration of this mid-nineteenth-century confidence exists than in the writers' on-going faith that a distinctive new literature will emerge in the region correlative with a growth in settlement and prosperity. From 1789 onwards, literary periodicals and newspapers cite the promise of their respective Nova Scotia, New Brunswick, or Prince Edward Island cultures. For Thomas Chandler Haliburton and Moses H. Perley, that promise included technological growth and a judicious development of natural resources. In 1798, Lieutenant Adam Allan of Fredericton saw a waterfall and rhapsodized in verse on its picturesque quality.[32] In 1835, Haliburton's Sam Slick saw a waterfall and wanted to put a carding mill, a circular saw, a turning lathe and a shingle machine on it.[33] The difference lies not just in convention. Haliburton was as appreciative of the beauty of his rural Maritime surroundings as anyone. Instead, it lies in the forward-looking, progressive nature of the vision entertained by many writers of the mid-century period. There is a strange "machine-in-the-garden" quality to Moses Perley's transformation of wilderness grandeur to gilded age growth in his 1840

---

27   Mrs. F. Beavan, *Life in the Backwoods of New Brunswick* (St. Stephen, New Brunswick, 1980 [1845]), p. 31.

28   Moodie, p. 237.

29   Oliver Goldsmith, "The Rising Village" in Douglas Daymond and Leslie Monkman, eds., *Literature in Canada*, Vol. 1 (Toronto, 1978), pp. 99-112.

30   Keefer, p. 35.

31   Thomas Chandler Haliburton, *The Old Judge or Life in a Colony* (Toronto, 1978 [1849]), p. 4. Quoted in Keefer, p. 35.

32   Adam Allan, "A Description of the Great Falls, of the River Saint John, in the Province of New Brunswick" in Daymond and Monkman, pp. 62-63.

33   Thomas Chandler Haliburton, *The Clockmaker* (Toronto, 1966 [1836]), p. 9.

fictional dream of a new "thriving village" rising out of the northern New Brunswick wilderness. Standing on a promontory in the centre of a vast forest, his persona sees in his "mind's eye" the church spire rising above the trees, hears the "clack" of the mill wheel by the "brawling stream," and senses the movement of carriages on newly-developed highways.[34] The vision fades, but not before it confirms for the reader that, much as Perley loves the primitivism and natural beauty of the wilderness informing his sporting sketches, he nonetheless sees the future in terms of development and change.

It is this note of "change" — what Charles G.D. Roberts calls the "hands of chance and change" — that begins to permeate Maritime literature in the late nineteenth century. Whether it is social, technological, or personal change that impels Roberts's persona to lament that the "Hands of chance and change have marred, or moulded, or broken,/Busy with spirit or flesh, all I most have adored," it is difficult to ascertain. As the essay "'A Past of Orchards'" in this collection notes, Roberts's decision at the end of "Tantramar Revisited" (1883) to "stay my steps and not go down to the marshland" — to cling to the "darling illusion"[35] that time and tranquillity have stood still on the Tantramar — indicates an escape into nostalgia and a boyhood past quite different in tone from the forward-looking energy of McCulloch or Haliburton. The "return" poems of Roberts and his cousin, Bliss Carman, carry with them a sense of loss, a yearning for a halcyon pastoral landscape of youth that contrasts the social and landscape writing of earlier Maritime literature. This sense of loss also enters the work of as strikingly different a writer as Joshua Slocum, the adventurous sailor from Brier Island, Nova Scotia, who inadvertently in his *Sailing Alone Around The World* (1899-1900) reveals a man rendered more obsolete than sorrowful by the "hands of chance and change." A master mariner, who in his prime owned and captained a windjammer, Slocum was passé by the 1890s when steam and the cut-throat economy of shipping had superceded men of sail. His rejection of a technological society emerges in his decision in 1895 to circumnavigate the world in a refurbished oyster sloop named the "Spray." In its own way a version of Roberts's "darling illusion," the "Spray" represents Slocum's clinging to a landscape, albeit a watery one, that still ensures him some sense of dignity and identity. Perhaps it is not inappropriate, therefore, that once the voyage of the "Spray" was over, once the hoop-la and the recognition of his

---

34 M.H. Perley, "Sporting Sketches From New Brunswick: No. 2. The Forest Fairies of the Milicetes," *The Sporting Review*, III (March 1840), pp. 191-96. For a discussion of Perley, see Gwendolyn Davies, "A Literary Study of Selected Periodicals From Maritime Canada: 1789-1872," (Ph.D. thesis, York University, 1979), pp. 136-48. For "machine in the garden", see Leo Marx, *The Machine in the Garden* (New York, 1964).

35 Charles G.D. Roberts, *The Collected Poems of Sir Charles G.D. Roberts* (Wolfville, Nova Scotia, 1985), pp. 78-79.

feat had subsided, and once the man and the boat had aged too long in harbour, the two set off on a last sea venture in 1909 from which they never returned.

From the deck of the "Spray" to the campus of King's College, Windsor, may seem an imaginative leap, but there is a sense in which both Slocum and Roberts reflect the spiritual restlessness, social upheaval, and *fin de siècle* quality of the late Victorian period in the Maritimes. Much has been written about the "flowering of Fredericton," the intellectual and cultural milieu from which the post-Confederation poets, Charles G.D. Roberts, Bliss Carman, Barry Stratton, and Francis Sherman emerged.[36] But of the "King's Circle" that developed around Roberts after he took up a post at the university in 1885, less has been said. Yet in this formative environment of the 1885-95 period, Roberts and Carman wrote some of their most evocative poetry of place about the Maritimes, in particular Roberts's "Tantramar Revisited" (1883) and "Ave" (1892), and Carman's "Low Tide on Grand Pré" (1887). Whereas Carman responded directly to the stimulus of the Minas Basin landscape, beginning what poet Charles Bruce described as Carman's "lifelong preoccupation with translating the changing face of nature,"[37] Roberts hearkened back to the other side of the Bay of Fundy and the boyhood images of the Tantramar Marsh where he lived until the age of fourteen. In the specificity of his Tantramar images, one senses from those years how Roberts learned to "see" the Marsh, both as a developing naturalist and as a young art student studying under the precise eye of painter, John Warren Gray, at Mount Allison.

In spite of Roberts's happy memories of the Tantramar, the King's years saw him satisfactorily surrounded by such young writers and artists as Goodridge Roberts, Robert Norwood, H.A. Cody, Sophie (Almon) Hensley, and the Prat sisters of Grand Pré. As well, poets and critics from abroad visited in the summers, even pitching tents on Roberts's lawn at Kingscroft to be present for the fellowship and literary conversation.[38] Such was Roberts's growing reputation at this juncture that a visit to Windsor to see him was an

---

36   See: A.G. Bailey, "Creative Moments In the Culture of the Maritime Provinces" in *Culture and Nationality* (Toronto, 1972), pp. 44-57; Malcolm Ross, "A Strange Aesthetic Ferment," in *The Impossible Sum of Our Traditions* (Toronto, 1986), pp. 27-42; and Carrie MacMillan, "Bishop Medley's Cathedral: Cultural Life In Early Confederation Fredericton" in Peter Thomas, ed. *The Red Jeep and Other Landscapes* (Fredericton, 1987), pp. 59-67.

37   Charles Bruce, "News Causes Deep Regret to People of Nova Scotia," *Telegraph Journal* (10 June 1929) in "Bliss Carman Memorial": a collection of newspaper clippings compiled by R.H. Hathaway, Hathaway Collection, University of New Brunswick. I wish to thank Dr. Terry Whalen of Saint Mary's University for drawing my attention to this item and to items in footnotes 43 & 44.

38   Maude Mary Clarke to Lorne Pierce, Wolfville, April 27 [1928], Lorne Pierce Papers, Box 3, "Correspondence 1928: A-H," Queen's University Archives.

appropriate hiatus in the North American tour of British critic and writer, Douglas Sladen, in 1893. *"O! Fortunati nimium sua si bona norint*, the people who live in this delicious country," he noted of the Annapolis Valley around Windsor: "No wonder that Roberts's nature-poems are so lovely; Charles Roberts, 'the Canadian Laureate' — Nova Scotia's link with the great world — lives in a pretty house in the croft behind the college.... He feels his seclusion from the great world, but living in the Arcadia of North America has given his poetry a certain aroma that one gets nowhere else in English verse."[39] It was part of Sladen's delight during this visit to wander over the marshes and fields of Windsor and Grand Pré with Roberts and Carman, for the cousins revelled in the countryside. As Maude Mary Clarke recalled years later: "The happiest part of Mr. Roberts' life at this time (I think) was when Carman came to Kingscroft.... Their thinking was so attuned to each other. They spend long afternoons on sunny days rambling over hill and pasture and at the tea table it would transpire that neither had spoken a word to the other. Could anything express more perfect harmony?"[40] However, the literary productivity and pleasure of those years was punctuated by the worry of supporting a growing family. In a letter to Lorne Pierce in 1928, Clarke remembered that "At Kingscroft — Dr. R. was the hardest-working man I've ever known. His college classes, literary work and his everlasting financing gave him little respite. The last-mentioned activity he invariably undertook, with great cheerfulness, but believe me it required great feats of engineering as his tired out-look testified, on his return."[41] To augment his professional and literary income, Roberts raised hens behind a high-stake fence in the backyard of Kingscroft, and early memories of family dinners are of the children's wiping plates and bowls with slices of bread and then tossing the crusts out of the dining room window to the waiting hens. Not only did this activity promote Roberts's money-making projects but it also saved the family the inconvenience of having to supply clean plates for the second course.[42] More frequently, however, the image associated with the two decades at King's is of a more literary, inspirational, or pastoral nature. "When Charles Roberts occupied the chair of English in King's College, Windsor, Nova Scotia," wrote Carman years later in 1921, "I was one of the foreign examiners in his subject and a frequent visitor in his home. Windsor is not far from Grand Pré, and I spent many happy vacations in the lovely Evangeline country. Of all the places I have known none is more enchanting in its peaceful and unspoiled serenity than Grand Pré was in those years. In

39 Douglas Sladen, *On the Cars and Off* (London, 1894), pp. 4-7.

40 Maude Mary Clarke to Lorne Pierce, Wolfville, March 31, 1928, Lorne Pierce Papers, Box 3, "Correspondence 1928: A-H," Queen's University Archives.

41 *Ibid.*

42 *Ibid.*

that bountiful land of great tides and wide meadows and comfortable quiet homes among miles of orchards, there was always something magical and charming which touched one with content and gladness. Or perhaps it is only because we were young and happy that the place must seem forever blessed." "That," adds Carman, acknowledging the sympathetic relationship between context and composition, "was when I was beginning to write verses, and the lines called 'Low Tide on Grand Pré' were composed in one of those summers."[43]

In spite of the inspirational beauty of the area, however, Sladen had identified a real problem for Roberts when he noted that the poet felt isolated from the wider world. Although *The Collected Letters of Charles G.D. Roberts* published by Goose Lane Editions in 1989 indicate the author's active correspondence with writers, editors, and journalists in America and Great Britain in the King's years, Roberts was nonetheless to leave his family and his teaching position in 1895 in search of greater scope for his restless energies. Neither he nor Carman was ever to forget his "King's Circle" connections, however, and the visit of both of them to Nova Scotia in 1928 just a year before Carman's death, coupled with their mutual commitment to the Song Fishermen group discussed in an essay in this collection, speaks of their reluctance to accept entirely the "hands of chance and change." When Bliss Carman died suddenly in New Canaan in June 1929, however, echoes of the "hands of chance and change" marring or moulding or breaking "all I most have adored" were again sounded. This time the loss can be heard in Roberts's terse press statement from Toronto: "To me he was not only the greatest of Canadian poets. He was also my best friend."[44]

Roy Daniells argues in the *Literary History of Canada* that Roberts never achieved the poetic heights of his contemporary, Archibald Lampman, but that as a man of letters, he generated enormous respect internationally and at home. Even in the King's years, this reputation was emerging. What Daniells calls "Roberts's sense of identity with the whole group of Canadian writers"[45] is clear in his correspondence to literary colleagues and in his generous support of aspiring authors, whether students or acquaintances. Not least among those protégés was the young Windsor resident, Sophie Almon, a descendant through Cotton Mather and Increase Mather of the intellectual traditions of New England and the great-granddaughter of Rebecca (Byles) Almon, one of Nova Scotia's liveliest eighteenth-century women letter writers. Whereas Rebecca (Byles) Almon had exhibited a very eighteenth-century sensibility when she protested that she was "by no means an advocate

---

43   Bliss Carman, "My Escape Into Poetry," *Saturday Night* (19 November 1921), p. 2.

44   "Pays Tribute," in "Bliss Carman Memorial."

45   Roy Daniells, "Lampman and Roberts," in Carl F. Klinck, *Literary History of Canada*, I (Toronto, 1976), pp. 414-15.

for a Womans ever exposing her Writings to the public Eye,"[46] her granddaughter represented a new generation of women when she wrote William Douw Lighthall of Montreal around 1890 seeking publication advice for her husband, H.A. Hensley, and herself as they set off on an international yacht trip.[47] The contributor of poems and volumes to such periodicals as *The Week, The Dominion Illustrated Monthly*, and *The Current*; a lecturer, journalist, and supporter of social activist causes in New York; and the author of collections of poetry and feminist essays, Sophie Almon Hensley represented the "New Women" who emerged on the Maritime literary landscape in the 1880s. Ann Ardis has pointed out that "New Women" writers in the 1880s and 1890s were often marginalized by critics and journalists, seen by many as contributing to the creation of a fictional woman who bore no relationship to actual women.[48] But there is no sense in Sophie Almon Hensley's poetry and prose of her inability to relate art to life. Her confidence in a new century is strong in an article in *The Arena* in 1899 as she notes: "The Suffragists have hewed and hacked their way through the solid phalanx of social opprobrium and selfish or indolent opposition; and the women of to-day, standing on the rising ground of a larger liberty and a more gracious freedom than would have been deemed possible in the past, give a grateful backward glance at their battle-scarred sisters ere they turn their expectant eyes upon the towering glory of a fuller enfranchisement."[49] Her poetry and prose hastened the day of that enfranchisement by their frank evocation of women's sexuality and ability to manage their own lives. *Love and the Woman of Tomorrow* (1913) developed themes from *The Arena* article by arguing that women should not feel pressured to marry, that those who wanted motherhood without marriage should not be discouraged, and that society, including the clergy, should develop more tolerance. Realistically discerning that much remained to be done in changing public attitudes, Hensley nonetheless portrayed a world in which women's courage would prevail:

> We are living in a man-made world, where men make laws not only for men but for women, where women are judged by men in the law-courts, are condemned to death by juries of men. Because quietness, humility and helplessness on the part of women made it easier for men

46   Rebecca Byles to her aunt, Halifax, 1 June 1785, Byles Papers, MG23, D6, Vol. III, National Archives of Canada.

47   Sophie M. Almon Hensley to W.D. Lighthall, Stellarton, n.d., Lighthall: O.S., Letters and Papers, undated, 1/1, McGill University Archives.

48   Ann L. Ardis, *New Women, New Novels* (New Brunswick, New Jersey, 1990), pp. 1-9 and pp. 12-13.

49   Almon Hensley, "The Society For The Study of Life," *The Arena* (November 1899), pp. 614-20.

to dominate them, to play with them, to subjugate them sexually, men have hindered the development of women individually, have stood between them and the expression of their powers. When one considers how women, in spite of the opposition of the sex that held the authority, that controlled the wealth, have made themselves heard, have invaded the professions and succeeded in them, have entered the arena of the business world and "made good," it only goes to show how tremendous is the strength, how indomitable is the courage, how wide and wise is the vision of the woman of to-day.[50]

Amongst Hensley's Maritime writing contemporaries, a similar, if sometimes more muted, note was struck. Novelists Alice and Susan Jones created strong women characters who travelled independently, had careers in art or journalism, and even got divorced. Anna Leonowens, of "Anna and the King of Siam" fame brought an eye for female injustice to her memoirs of the Far East and worked with Halifax women in the late nineteenth century on a variety of suffragist and social causes. And Marshall Saunders, often remembered primarily for children's animal stories like *Beautiful Joe*, employed both the speaker's platform and her fiction to further the educational and social role of women. In *The Story of the Gravelys. A Tale for Girls* (1903), her protagonist Berty Gravely fights city hall to get a playground for the poor, denounces marriage as "slavery to some man,"[51] and warns a would-be assailant that "a gymnasium-trained girl like myself could knock you about easily."[52] Her vision of the life of poor working girls ends in the proclamation, "I don't see why the poor don't organize. They are meeker than I would be."[53] While there are conservative dimensions to Saunders's feminism and a suggestion in *The Story of the Gravelys* that Berty will shortly succumb to love and marriage, the author nonetheless created in a spirited protagonist like Berty the voice of change and conscience that she and other women writers from Nova Scotia saw as essential to society's well-being.

While essays in this collection such as "Dearer Than His Dog" explore representative writers and moments in women's literary history in the Maritimes, much research remains to be done in this area and in others to complete any full study of the region's literary development. Included in this is the influence of one generation of writers on another, for the homogeneity of Maritime society frequently brought publications and writers to the attention of one another. The *Acadian Magazine* of 1826-28 and *The British*

---

50   Almon Hensley, *Love and The Woman of Tomorrow* (London, 1913), p. 243.

51   Marshall Saunders, *The Story of The Gravelys* (London, 1905 [1903]), p. 243.

52   *Ibid.*, pp. 199-200.

53   *Ibid.*, p. 234.

North American Magazine of 1831 acknowledged the precedent of *The Nova-Scotia Magazine* of 1789-92; the Club group of 1828 spoke warmly of the satirical sketches of McCulloch's 1821-23 Stepsure letters; Douglas Huyghue wrote his 1841-43 novel, *Argimou. A Legend of the Micmac* while a friend of Indian Commissioner and sporting sketch writer, Moses Perley; Sophie (Almon) Hensley inspired a Roberts poem in the 1880s while also enjoying Roberts's sponsorship; Charles Bruce was befriended at Mount Allison in the 1920s by established writers, Robert Norwood and Frank Parker Day; Ernest Buckler, working his way through university in the 1930s, received books and encouragement from Archibald MacMechan; and David Adams Richards, studying at St. Thomas University in the 1970s, enjoyed the literary friendship of Alden Nowlan. The pattern of continuity, of inter-action, and of inter-texuality has continued. "Charles G.D./Roberts, pince-nez and tails, flies/like an angel by Stanley Spencer over/this place"[54] notes Douglas Lochhead in *High Marsh Road. Lines for a Diary* as he exhibits the same eye for the painterly, the visual, as Roberts himself. The marsh, the sky, the horizon, the wind reverberate for Lochhead. Here, in the diary entry for September 1, are images of "Colville's Crow" mounting "higher higher./the silver spoon is fast in the beak." There, on November 16, are "the corners/of Christopher Pratt's windows." Before him at Jolicure on November 27 is the grave of poet John Thompson, one of "the dead who sing": "only the flag on my/friend's plot waves. there is the/murmur of his voice. word after/word. there is no forgetting John." It "is/good to have such footsteps,"[55] he muses in an earlier entry about Roberts, and out of this interaction of visual and poetic responses to the broad beauty of the landscape comes the diary entry for October 19: "this is my place." In affirming place, the Lochhead speaker gives climax to more than 200 years of Maritime literary voice. Or, as Harry Thurston, a poet of another generation, puts it: "Yet it is as if our fathers/our grandfathers had never left./...Can you see a Cape Island boat/without wanting to steer it to her source?"[56]

Steering to our sources. It is the hope that this is what the essays in this collection begin to do. Much voyaging has been done. Much of the journey remains.

---

54 Douglas Lochhead, *High Marsh Road. Lines for a Diary* (Toronto: 1980), October 19.

55 *Ibid.*, October 9.

56 Harry Thurston, *Clouds Flying Before the Eye* (Fredericton, 1985), p. 10.

Persona in Planter Journals

In *His Majesty's Yankees* by Thomas Raddall, the Planter merchant, Simeon
Perkins, is depicted as "unheroic, uneasy, un-everything."[1] The portrait is
anything but flattering, but the inspiration for it lies not in Raddall's creative
imagination but in the private journals maintained by Perkins from 1766 to
1812, the year in which he died in his adopted home of Nova Scotia. A native
of Norwich, Connecticut, Simeon Perkins had immigrated to Liverpool on the
south shore of the province in May 1762 only three years after Governor
Charles Lawrence had issued warrants to survey the township. Beginning as a
dealer in lumber and fish, Perkins went on to become a prominent property
owner, merchant, farmer, mill operator, shipbuilder and Atlantic trader, as
well as a member of the Legislative Assembly, a Justice of the Courts, a
Judge of Probate and a Colonel Commandant of the Militia for Queens
County. By the time of his death, he was described as a "father" to the town
of Liverpool, known, as his obituary pointed out, for "great wisdom, general
knowledge, piety and benevolence, and uncommon usefulness."[2]

"Uncommon usefulness" is an unsentimental attribution for someone to
bear in death as in life; yet a reading of the five volumes of Simeon Perkins's
diary published by the Champlain Society reveals a persona consistent with
The Weekly Chronicle's assessment of Liverpool's leading citizen. Writing in
his journal more frequently after war broke out in 1775 than before, Perkins
records what he has seen and done and heard. There is nothing introspective
or analytical about his entries. His journal is intended to document financial
matters, ships leaving harbour, occurrences in the meeting house, weather
conditions, or visitations of family and friends. However, it becomes
something more because of the historical events in which Perkins is caught
up. "Experiencing life as a graduated succession of changes is an absolute
prerequisite for writing a journal,"[3] argues Robert Fothergill in *Private
Chronicles: A Study of English Diaries*, and in Perkins's case, these changes
were precipitated not so much by the domestic crises and financial
transactions that punctuated his everyday life as by the political events
between 1766 and 1812 that drew him willy-nilly into the fray, expanded his
social and business horizons, and brought new stimuli to the town he had
helped to nourish. Beginning as a personal recorder of mundane matters,
Perkins was to become a self-appointed chronicler of his community in a
period of enormous social change.

---

1   Thomas H. Raddall, *His Majesty's Yankees* (Toronto, 1977 [1942]), p. 43.

2   C.B. Fergusson, ed., *The Diary of Simeon Perkins, 1804-1812* (Toronto, 1978), p. liii.

3   Robert A. Fothergill, *Private Chronicles: A Study of English Diaries* (London, 1924), p. 14.

The catalyst for many of his observations came with his increasing role of responsibility within the township, for public affairs had become part of his private domain. Concurrent with Simeon's growing prominence within the town, however, was the outbreak first of the American Revolution, then of the Napoleonic Wars, and later of the War of 1812. In all of these cases, one senses that the Simeon Perkins of the journals shrinks from a breakdown of rational order and all that it implies. Thomas Raddall suggests Perkins's state of bewilderment when he compares him to "a sad little saw-whet owl"[4] when he is faced with the choices of the American Revolution. Yet, seemingly unhindered by any kind of active imagination, Simeon was able to initiate militia offensives and to document the social, economic, and religious impact of the times on townspeople like himself living on the sea-lanes of the conflict. It is this unvarnished quality that Raddall recognized as a valuable resource in Perkins's journals when he first read them in the 1930s and it is for this reason that Raddall's fictional treatment of Liverpool's Strang family in *His Majesty's Yankees* strikes true in idiom, domestic realism and historical detail.

While Simeon Perkins's journals grew out of his personal experience, they also represent part of the greater impulse toward journal writing that flowered in the seventeenth and eighteenth centuries. Pepys' famous *Diary* maintained from 1660-69 had set a standard as a personal record of the times, and in the very year that Perkins removed to Liverpool from Connecticut, James Boswell had begun his *London Journal* by vowing to preserve the "many things that would otherwise be lost in oblivion."[5] Yet there was a marked difference between Boswell's journal and Pepys's, for Boswell was preoccupied less with events than with his self-conscious role in them. Boswell, as Fothergill points out, is more egocentric than is Pepys, who desires only "to cherish the events of each day, not because they are the theatre for his latest manifestation, but because they are what actually happened and as such deserve to be acknowledged."[6] Boswell creates a persona satisfactory to himself in a way unknown to either Pepys or Perkins. There are few revelations of self in Simeon Perkins's documentation of events, and when he does allow opinion to intrude into his record of wind and weather, the revelations are not inconsistent with the plain, blunt man who has been emerging: "I have been applied to for my approbation" of a dance, he wrote on 12 January 1797; "I think it rather premature in such a Young Settlement, and Considering the late frowns of Providence in the death of several of our young men, & others missing, and the threatening aspects of

---

4   Raddall, *His Majesty's Yankees*, p. 6.

5   Fothergill, *Private Chronicles*, p. 78.

6   *Ibid.*, p. 71.

public affairs, I think it highly Improper at this time, whether it might be in other Situations & Circumstances."[7]

Elsewhere his observations can be more personal, focusing as he grew older as much on the affairs of his family as on the progress of the settlement. Typical of a rare glimpse into the sense of obligation he felt toward his children is the placing of his daughter Mary in a Halifax boarding school at the cost of £35 in October 1804. "It is expensive," he notes, "but I think it my duty to give my children what Education I can, and this daughter acquiring Something may give the others an Opportunity to gain Something from her advantage."[8] Such insights into Perkins's character reveal enough of a persona to elevate the diary beyond the level of mere memoranda.

In this sense, Perkins's journal is far more interesting than are the Planter journals of the Reverend John Seccombe and his daughter of Chester with their litany of meals and visitations respectively. The Seccombe journals reveal life led day-to-day in 1761, illustrating in the very narrowness of their references the limitations of living in a community less strategic to the sea-lanes than was Liverpool. Moreover, the pattern of the Seccombe diaries suggests an exercise in personal documentation. On "Satterday," 21 November 1761, for example, the Reverend Mr. Seccombe noted: "Fair, cool — Pork & Cabbage Turnep &c for dinner — P.M. went with Mr Bridge to ye mill, & to view a Lot. Supped on Moose Stakes, dry'd meat. Indians brought in wild Fowl. Bever &c."[9] In the Perkins diaries, by contrast, there is the very real sense that Simeon is writing more of a record and from time to time will turn back to the pages of his journal to check an incident or a date in the 46 years of his recording. As Alan Young has noted in his book, *Thomas H. Raddall*, there are striking parallels between Perkins's diary-keeping and that of Sumter Larabee, a central figure in Raddall's *The Wedding Gift and Other Stories*. "The Diary of Sumter Larabee" was the "journal of a realist," he quotes Raddall, "written with an obsession for present facts and the deuce with past or future. Sumter seldom followed up an incident or looked back to compare anything but the weather or the date of last year's turnip planting."[10] Such seems to be the situation of Simeon Perkins whose sense of history was practical and whose future was always in the hands of God.

Of all the journals emerging from the Planter experience, it is those that probe the individual's relationship with God that best exemplify the qualities of introspection and analysis associated with the development of a persona in

---

7   D.C. Harvey, ed., *The Diary of Simeon Perkins, 1780-1789* (Toronto, 1958), p. xxxviii.

8   C.B. Fergusson, ed., *The Diary of Simeon Perkins, 1804-1812* (Toronto, 1979), p. 70.

9   "The Diary of the Reverend John Seccombe," *Report of the Public Archives of Nova Scotia* (Halifax, 1959), Appendix B, pp. 18-47, 240. See also "Memoranda of Leading Events by a member of the Seccombe Family," PANS, MG 1, vol. 797C, No. 2.

10   Alan Young, *Thomas H. Raddall* (Boston, 1983), p. 79.

journal literature. As Steven Kagle has pointed out in *American Diary Literature, 1620-1799*, the spiritual journey occupied a central place in colonial America. Usually employing a standardized rhetoric and modelled after celebrated examples, the spiritual journey "allowed its author to find a pattern which could reveal the truth of the past and plan the direction of the future."[11] Particularly in Puritan diaries were the conventions of self-examination, self-abasement and dramatic conversion developed. For Puritans, salvation was an arbitrary thing dependent on the will of God, and the maintenance of a religious register was not only a way of justifying one's conduct but also a process of documenting one's path to election or grace. In a sense, then, as Kagle and others imply, the spiritual journal was a statement against despair, a form of confessional which the Puritan or Calvinist would construct in the spiritual isolation that went with his or her self-analysis. Casting back to his youth in his spiritual journey, Henry Alline of Falmouth, Nova Scotia, remembered in the 1780s that "God...gave me a sense of my lost and undone condition in a great degree: fearing almost anything that I saw, that it was against me; commissioned from God to call me away, and I was unprepared: I was even afraid of trees falling on me, when I was in the woods, and in a time of thunder would expect the next flash of lightening was commissioned to cut me off. Thus I was one of the unhappiest creatures that lived on earth; and would promise and vow, in time of danger, that I would leave all my carnal mirth and vain company, and that I would never rest until I had found rest in my soul."[12]

Alline's expression of fear and unworthiness is a stock convention in Puritan and Calvinist journals and finds repetition in the spiritual journals of two other Planter writers, Jonathan Scott of Chebogue and Mary Coy Bradley of Gagetown and Saint John. For both Alline and Bradley, this fear coloured their childhood years, so that Alline would pray even on his way to school "that this angry God would not send me to hell,"[13] and Mary Bradley would agonize, "how can I dwell in flames of fire and brimstone, through an endless eternity!"[14] Entering a covenant with the Lord dispelled that fear for both authors, but their pre-covenant terror is more rhetorical than chilling because of the retrospective nature of their journals. Alline's work was begun during his ministry in the late 1770s and, at the time of his death in 1784 was left to

---

11   Steven A. Kagle, *American Diary Literature, 1620-1799* (Boston, 1979), p. 29-57. For a discussion of gender in conversion narratives, see Susan Juster, "'In a Different Voice': Male and Female Narratives of Religious Conversion in Post Revolutionary America," *American Quarterly*, No. 41 (March 1989), pp. 34-62.

12   Henry Alline, *The Life and Journal of Rev. Mr. Henry Alline* (Boston, 1806), p. 29.

13   *Ibid.*, p. 4.

14   Mary Bradley, *A Narrative of the Life and Christian Experience of Mrs. Mary Bradley* (Boston, 1849), p. 28.

circulate privately in manuscript form, finally reaching publication in Boston in 1806.

Bradley's work was also destined for a public audience, becoming one of many Wesleyan-Methodist spiritual records published in the mid-nineteenth century in the wake of diaries by John Wesley, George Whitefield and others. While intensely focused on the routine events of Mrs. Bradley's Christian life, the *Narrative of...Mrs. Mary Bradley* does project into the litany of Methodist religious records the perspective of a woman who wanted to play anything but a passive role in the profession of her faith. "I always heard that women had nothing to do in public, respecting religious exercises," she noted early in her journal, "and that it was absolutely forbidden in the scriptures for a woman to pray in public, or to have anything to say in the church of God. Under the consideration of those things, I felt much shame and confusion and knew not how to endure it."[15] Elsewhere in her journal she chafes under the social and marriage bonds that require sublimation of her opinions to those of her first husband: "But soon I found that, being his wife, I was bound by law to yield obedience to the requirements of my husband; and when he enforced obedience, and showed marks of resentment if his wishes were not met, I was tempted with anger and felt a spirit of resentment arise in my heart and retaliating expressions come into my mind...."[16] As Margaret Conrad has pointed out in an introduction to Mrs. Bradley's narrative in *Atlantis* in 1981, her authorship offers glimpses into the social and legal position of women in the Planter community and reveals something of the work patterns of such women in rural areas of the Maritimes.[17] However, the overall narrowness of Mary Bradley's interests restricts the emergence of a distinct persona in her journal. Only when she recalls her childhood in Gagetown or describes the early years of her marriage is there a glimpse of the human being behind the stylized rhetoric of the spiritual diary. On the whole, Mary Bradley's journal conforms to established patterns and rarely offers those touches of domestic originality that emerge when she pauses in her weeding to compare herself to a good seed choked by weeds in the garden of Christ.[18]

It is in their inability to transcend the conventions of their genre that many of the spiritual journalists fail in literary terms. The literary critic, as Robert Fothergill has pointed out, "is concerned with that work in which the impulsion to articulate the self has precipitated discovery of a fresh organization of the form's potential. The most remarkable displays of this

15 *Ibid.*, p. 50.

16 *Ibid.*, p. 106.

17 Margaret Conrad, "Mary Bradley's Reminiscences: A Domestic Life in Colonial New Brunswick," *Atlantis*, 7, 1 (Fall 1981), p. 92.

18 Mary Bradley, *A Narrative*, p. 43.

discovery we call genius, and the diary indeed has its geniuses."[19] Amongst the spiritual journalists writing from the Planter experience, there seem to be few with this spark, for profession of faith rather than literary self-consciousness is both their intent and their preoccupation. The range is not wide, and even in the hands of so charismatic a figure as Henry Alline, the spiritual diary fails to reveal a persona so much as a vocation. This being said, it cannot be denied that Alline demonstrates a flair for dramatic presentation and an energy of phrasing that circumvent some of the limitations of the spiritual diary form. While honouring the same conventions as his spiritual colleagues (the terror of religion in childhood, the isolation of the unsaved soul, the revelation and covenant with God, the mission to carry the message), Alline can transform language into a powerful crescendo of euphony, rhythm, and harmony as he describes himself, "groaning under mountains of death, wading through storms of sorrow, racked with distressing fears, and crying to an unknown God for help...."[20] As George Rawlyk has pointed out, Alline's power with language annoyed his Congregationalist opponent, Jonathan Scott, who saw Alline's work as "interspersed with Poetry calculated to excite and raise the Passions of the Reader, especially the young, ignorant and inconsistent, who are influenced more by the sound and Gingle of the words, then by solid Sentences and rational and scriptural Ideas of divine and eternal Things."[21] Moreover, as a journeyer as well as a journalist, Alline had an opportunity to meet new people, see new areas and hear new arguments. This range of constantly shifting sights, sounds and experiences enlivens the pace of his diary in a way denied the home-bound Mary Bradley or the congregation-tied Jonathan Scott. Steven Kagle has argued that it was often the diaries of itinerant Methodists that focused "outward to the world, giving a valuable picture of their world."[22] Alline's case is similar. The travel pattern of his journal expands it beyond the conventional structure of many spiritual records and enables Alline to explore religious questions within a wider and more interesting social context. In the main part of his journal, he is not isolated physically or spiritually as he was before he made his covenant with God. Rather he functions on a broad geographical stage where his personal journey and his relations with others coalesce in a book designed to illuminate the lives of many.

As revealing as individual Planter journals can be about the social, political and religious lives of the speakers and their communities, there is little in the conventionalized language and format of most of these records to warrant their being called "literature" in the creative or imaginative sense. Thus, to

---

19 Fothergill, *Private Chronicles*, p. 12.

20 Alline, *The Life and Journal*, pp. 34-35.

21 George A. Rawlyk, ed., *The Sermons of Henry Alline* (Hantsport, 1986), p. 28.

22 Kagle, *American Diary Literature*, p. 51.

speak of a Planter literature is to speak of a Planter body of writing, for there is nothing of the development to be found in later journals where literary self-consciousness made the persona assume a stance akin to that of a fictional character. In their dedication to fulfil their tasks, the Planter writers noted others as characters in the play of life (both Perkins and Bradley describe the visits of Alline, for example), but themselves only as vehicles (Alline wanted to be a mouth for God). It is left to the later generations of Thomas Raddall, Greg Cook and Douglas Lochhead, amongst the creative writers, and Michael Miller amongst the composers, to breathe imaginative life into the earnest personae who emerge from the Planter journals of Perkins, Seccombe, Alline and Bradley.[23]

---

23 As has been mentioned, Thomas Raddall adapted his knowledge of Simeon Perkins and his diary into literary dramatizations in *His Majesty's Yankees, At The Tide's Turn and Other Stories*, and *The Wedding Gift and Other Stories*. Maritime poets, Greg Cook and Douglas Lochhead, have been interested in making Alline the subject of poems. Douglas Lochhead's "Homage to Henry Alline," was read at Acadia University in October 1990. A concert version of Michael Miller's opera on Alline was performed at Mount Allison University in February 1990.

Consolation to Distress:
Loyalist Literary Activity in the Maritimes

The Loyalist migration into the Maritime Provinces has often been examined for its social, economic, and political impact, but it is also to the Loyalists that literary historians must turn in any discussion of creative activity in the area during the early years of its cultural development. Among the approximately 30,000 refugees settling in the region were a number of the most active literary figures of the Revolutionary War period, including such well-respected Tory satirists as Jonathan Odell, Jacob Bailey, and Joseph Stansbury, and a number of lesser-known occasional writers like Mather Byles, Jr., Roger Viets, Joshua Wingate Weeks, and Deborah How Cottnam. Bringing with them a sophistication of literary experience and a taste for lyric and satiric writing hitherto unknown in the region, these authors were part of a wider Loyalist cultural phenomenon that saw the founding of schools and classical colleges, the endorsement of theatrical performances, the development of newspapers and printing shops, the organization of agricultural and reading societies, and the writing of polite literature as part of the fabric of conventional society. Looking to their old life as a measure of the new, Loyalist exiles in the Maritimes did much to develop the expectations, structures, and standards of taste necessary for the growth of a literary environment. Although economics, geography, politics, and personal differences militated against their founding a literary movement between 1776 and 1814 or leaving behind an identifiable literary tradition, the Loyalists did illustrate the imaginative and cultural possibilities awaiting a later, more securely-established generation of writers. When an indigenous literature finally did begin to develop, first in the columns of newspapers like *The Acadian Recorder* (founded 1813) and then in the periodicals of the 1820s and 1830s, the debt of that next, native-born generation to the Loyalists and their cultural institutions was both obvious and acknowledged.

Of all the Loyalist writers who came to the Maritime Provinces after 1775, the Reverend Jacob Bailey and the Reverend Jonathan Odell were the most prolific in output and the most enduring in reputation. Particularly effective in a war-time climate where satire dominated as a literary form and where a sense of immediacy heightened the passion of ridicule,[1] Bailey and Odell shared with other Loyalists a sense of bitterness and betrayal after the cessation of hostilities in 1783. Of the two, Bailey was the most tenacious in continuing to explore political themes in his writing after leaving American soil. A Church of England clergyman from Pownalborough, Maine, who had moved to Nova Scotia in 1779 to escape persecution, Bailey turned

---

1 Bruce Granger, *Political Satire in the American Revolution* (Ithaca, 1960), pp. 5-7.

increasingly to the Hudibrastic conventions of Samuel Butler to reduce and caricature his republican subjects. For Bailey, writing poetry and prose was a form of consolation, a way of re-articulating his moral vision in the face of folly and insanity. "When I am disappointed, harassed or chagrined," he wrote Samuel Peters in 1780, "I immediately revenge myself upon the fathers of the rebellion."[2] Thus, in such poems as "The Factious Demagogue" or "The Character of a Trimmer" written during the war years, he lashed out at the equivocation, irrationality, and stupidity of the rebels and their political philosophy. Although the world as he knew it was disintegrating, Bailey was able to enshrine in his writing the old verities that gave moral and social direction to his life.

After 1783 when the Tory cause had finally collapsed, Bailey ceased flagellating the perpetrators of the war and began to focus instead on themes of encroachment and betrayal, particularly directing his wrath against American Methodism and the hypocrisy he perceived in the post-war Loyalist camp. Poems such as his Hudibrastic narrative "The Adventures of Jack Ramble, The Methodist Preacher" (c.1787-1795) reflected Bailey's sense of frustration over the spread of levelling principles into Nova Scotia, and a short satire on the Reverend Jonathan Odell revealed his sensitivity to the shifts in personal loyalty that were beginning to take place among the post-war exiles. An admirer of Odell's Revolutionary War satires, Bailey felt aggrieved when his fellow clergyman visited Annapolis Royal en route to his new post as Provincial Secretary of New Brunswick and failed to pay his social respects to either Bailey or his former Loyalist compatriots. "I suppose you are sufficiently informed that your worthy Secretary of New Brunswick was formerly a clergyman and Missionary of Burlington in the Jersies with a salary of fifty pounds a year," Bailey wrote to Henry Barlow Brown of St. Andrews on 31 January 1785, "and in his progress from Halifax to the seat of his appointment he was at Annapolis several days at which time there resided at my house two daughters of Dr. Seabury, Mr. Campbell of Burlington, clerk of your Supreme Court, Mr. Cutler a Merchant and his Lady a daughter of Col. Hicks, all of these had been his fellow passengers — and yet this newly exalted being never once called at the house to look upon his former brother, or his ship-mates — three of whom had been his most intimate acquaintance." "To amuse the Ladies," added Bailey, "and to soften the chagrin we all felt at being denied a visit from this dignified priest, I wrote a couple of poems — the former it is not prudent to insert — but the other in

---

2. Jacob Bailey to Samuel Peters, 26 November 1780, Samuel Peters Papers, Church Historical Society, Austin, Texas. Also quoted in Thomas B. Vincent, "Keeping the Faith: The Poetic Development of Jacob Bailey, Loyalist," *Early American Literature*, XII (Spring 1979), p. 8.

the same kind of measure as his poem on Dr. Franklin I here produce."[3] The resulting parody of Odell's "Inscription for a Curious Chamber Stove" detailed how Bailey had "waited in vain to behold/ Such a favorite man of my tribe." The snub was followed by salutary if rueful reflections, causing the poet-speaker to draw the bitter conclusion — "I have learnt that those mortals who soar/ aloft on the wings of ambition/ disdain their importance to lower/ to friends of their former condition."[4]

In spite of the trenchant quality of satires such as this one, it is likely that the private nature of its circulation prevented Bailey's work from having a broad influence on public taste in the Maritimes.[5] Ironically, Jonathan Odell, that "man of my tribe" whom Bailey had grown to despise, was to be more conspicuously and frequently associated with Maritime satire in the late eighteenth and early nineteenth centuries than was Bailey. It was Odell, "the leading Tory satirist of the American Revolution," Alfred Bailey argues, "whose literary propensities helped indirectly to form the tradition in which Carman and Roberts were nurtured."[6] It was also Jonathan Odell to whom Ray Palmer Baker turned as the literary progenitor of Thomas Chandler Haliburton and his circle during Nova Scotia's intellectual awakening in the 1820s and the 1830s.[7] Using "the heroic couplet with a dash and vigour attained by no other Revolutionary writer except Freneau," noted Baker in *A History of English-Canadian Literature to the Confederation*, Jonathan Odell "stamped his conservative ideas and his satiric methods on Canadian literature."[8] Yet such a claim for Odell poses problems for any modern analysis of the poet's influence, since even a cursory examination of the availability and content of Odell's poetry after he removed to New Brunswick belies Baker's assumption that Odell had a stylistic and philosophical impact on a successive generation of writers. Less than a dozen of Odell's poems were published in provincial newspapers after 1785 and his verses did not become available in book form until 1857-60 when *The Loyalist Poetry of the Revolution* and *The Loyal Verses of Joseph Stansbury and Doctor Jonathan Odell* were published in limited editions in the United States.[9] Moreover, his

---

3   Jacob Bailey to Henry Barlow Brown, 31 January 1785, "Places: Annapolis Royal," Fort Anne Papers, reel 1, letter 17, pp. 92-95, Public Archives of Nova Scotia (PANS).

4   *Ibid.*

5   Thomas B. Vincent, *Narrative Verse Satire in Maritime Canada, 1779-1814* (Ottawa, 1978), p. 3, n. 10.

6   Alfred Bailey, "Creative Moments in the Culture of the Maritime Provinces" in G.A. Rawlyk, ed., *Historical Essays on the Atlantic Provinces* (Toronto, 1967), p. 239.

7   Ray Palmer Baker, *A History of English-Canadian Literature to the Confederation* (Cambridge, Mass., 1920), p. 71.

8   *Ibid.*, p. 28.

9   Winthrop Sargent, ed., *The Loyalist Poetry of the Revolution* (Philadelphia, 1857) and *The Loyal Verses of Joseph Stansbury and Doctor Jonathan Odell* (Albany, 1860).

poems after 1785 tended to be domestic and patriotic in nature, becoming satirical again only in 1812 when the American invasion of the Canadas re-awakened the spirit of outrage that had provoked his political writing during the Revolution.

What Jonathan Odell, Jacob Bailey, and other Loyalist writers did do was to introduce into the Maritime region and into Maritime literature a body of active and educated authors who regarded the composition of poetry and prose not only as a pleasant avocation but also as a social grace reflecting the standards of taste and sensibility of a cultured society. That many of these writers were Anglican clerics was of significance, for the American clergy had exerted considerable influence over their nation's literary life in the seventeenth and eighteenth centuries.[10] Many Tory clergy merely transferred this relationship and influence into the Maritimes when they left the United States, reaffirming through their authorship their sense of traditional values. They did not perceive the writer to be an agent of innovation or change. "The role of the poet at this stage in Maritime literature," as Tom Vincent has argued, "was not to explore or create uncharted literary worlds, but to establish a cultural base that 'meant something' to the people for whom he wrote. These people were trying to establish themselves in a variety of ways, and, consciously or unconsciously, the poet worked to do his part."[11]

Nowhere was the public role of poetry and the poet better illustrated than in the Reverend Roger Viets' "Annapolis-Royal." Appearing first in pamphlet form in Halifax and then on 12 August 1788 in *The Halifax Gazette*, the poem opens with a conventional image of order and harmony. "The King of Rivers" flows languorously through "fair" and "verdant" banks decked in "gayest Cloathing of perpetual Green." As the Annapolis River reaches the sea, this marriage achieves fruition in the vision of Annapolis-Royal, that "Royal Settlement," "washed" by the river, "blest" by Heaven, and "dear" to the poet. The imagery throughout the first part of the poem is pastoral, reinforcing the sense of a harmonious plan of divinity informing this world and offering the stability on which "a newborn race" could be "rear'd by careful Hands."[12]

The progress of Viets' poem was designed to complement the vision of society projected by the poet in the opening, pastoral sections. The village is a

10 Emory Elliott, *Revolutionary Writers. Literature and Authority in the New Republic, 1725-1810* (New York, 1982), pp. 26-28. For further references to the role of the Tory clergy in Nova Scotia, see Arthur Hamilton Wentworth Eaton, *The Church of England in Nova Scotia and the Tory Clergy of the Revolution* (New York, 1891) and Judith Fingard, *The Anglican Design in Loyalist Nova Scotia, 1783-1816* (London, 1972).

11 Thomas B. Vincent, "Eighteenth Century Poetry in Maritime Canada: Problems of Approach — A Research Report" in Kenneth MacKinnon, ed., *Atlantic Provinces Literature Colloquium* (Saint John, 1977), p. 18.

12 Roger Viets, *Annapolis-Royal* (1788: rpt. Kingston, 1979), pp. 1, 2, 4.

model of eighteenth-century order where "The Streets, the Buildings, Gardens, all concert/ To please the Eye, to gratify the Heart." Within the context of this town plan, "decent mansions" rise, "deck'd with moderate Cost,/ of honest Thrift, and gen'rous Owners boast." Hard work, marriage, procreation, and death all unfold within the confines of this community, reinforcing a vision of the future when the "Newborn race" "Thr'o numerous Ages thus they'll happy move/ In active Bus'ness, and in chastest Love." Two-thirds of the way through "Annapolis-Royal," the writer effects a synthesis of pastoral and town imagery in anticipation of the claims and the purpose of his poem: a revelation of the Divine power behind the rural and social harmony just described. His symbol of this power evolves naturally from the architectural references provided earlier in the poem, for the eye is now invited to move from the "gardens," "streets," and "decent mansions" of the town landscape to the "Spire majestic" rearing "it's [sic] solemn Vane" over the community. Here, under man's symbol of God's order and benevolence, the rector marshals his spiritual forces and sets an example for his "flock" by eschewing "pomp," "pride," and the "empty joys of Sense." In the hierarchical structure of the community where he represents both church and state, the rector is the one who most fully appreciates the significance of the "celestial" choir that raises its voice to God under the "Spire majestic." In an image consistent with Viets' eighteenth-century social vision, the poet envisages a band of "Youths and Virgins fair,/ Rank'd in due Order," harmonizing their strains until "By those harmonious Sounds such Rapture's giv'n,/ Their loud Hosannas waft the Soul to Heav'n:/ The fourfold Parts, in one bright Center meet,/ To form the blessed Harmony complete." The poem ends, then, on a note of harmony and order, proffering a vision of stability and growth if civilization honours certain values and social conventions.[13]

Although "Annapolis-Royal" can be read as a topographical and inspirational poem,[14] it was in many respects a political poem as well. Viets, Anglican rector of Digby and a Loyalist from Simsbury, Connecticut, reaffirmed in his verse the values which the Loyalist elite had sought to protect. The world he presents is ordered, stable, hierarchical, and conservative. At the very heart of it is the Anglican Church, a symbol of God and the Crown. In the aftermath of the Revolution, British policy endorsed placing Church of England clergymen "in every strategic locality, to hold aloft the torch of civilization, to become a little centre of culture, and a recruiting agency for schools."[15] In a sense, Viets and his poem fulfilled that official aim. In the midst of exile and financial exigency, the rector offered quiet reassurance that

---

13   *Ibid.*, pp. 3-6.

14   Thomas B. Vincent, "Introduction" to *ibid.*, p. v.

15   D.C. Harvey, "The Intellectual Awakening of Nova Scotia" in Rawlyk, ed., *Historical Essays on the Atlantic Provinces*, p. 105.

the refugees' world would be rebuilt. "We and our Cause were ruined together," Viets observed in a sermon on "Brotherly Love" delivered to his Digby congregation in 1789: "So [God] in his all-wise Providence, for Reasons unknown to Us, gave Us up, like Holy Job, to Affliction & Distress; the just and wise tho' unsearchable Providence of God has placed Us in a Neighbourhood together; in which Situation, altho' We want some of the Conveniences, & many of the Luxuries of this [world], yet We enjoy all the Spiritual Privileges that any People ever *did* or ever *can* enjoy."[16] By striking an affirmative note in his sermon, Viets was in fact upholding the "torch of civilization" that had been threatened by war and exile. By writing and distributing "Annapolis-Royal," he was also representing that "centre of culture" that Church and State saw as essential in reinforcing British values in the Maritimes.

In spite of the positive note struck by Viets in his sermon and his poem, he identified a very real problem for the Loyalists when he observed that "We want some of the Conveniences, & many of the Luxuries of this [world]." Looking back on his childhood in Nova Scotia from the vantage point of the 1860s, the Reverend James Cuppaidge Cochran, the son of a Loyalist, recalled that even in the late 1790s and the early 1800s, "We had no reading rooms — no lectures — no social gatherings for mental improvement — no performer to delight the ear and refine the taste by his admirable readings — no libraries except two filled with such things as Mrs. Radcliffe's romances, about haunted castles, mysterious knockings, after reading which, one would cover up the head and be afraid to go to sleep — We had nothing in short to elevate and improve."[17] Cochran's recollections find reinforcement in the letters, diaries, and documents of many Loyalists who came into the region between 1783 and 1789. Writing to Lord Hawkesbury a few years after the war, Charles Inglis similarly noted: "On my arrival at Halifax soon after I was appointed Bishop of this new Diocese in 1787, I found the country destitute of the means of education — there was not even a good Grammar-school in the whole of the province."[18] "Nothing but wilderness," was the way Walter Bates put it on arriving in New Brunswick in 1783 — "Nothing but wilderness before our eyes; the women and children *did not refrain from tears!*"[19]

---

16 Roger Viets, "On Brotherly Love," Sermons: Reverend Roger Viets, Lawrence Collection (Ward Chipman), MG 23, D1, series 1, Vol. 14, Public Archives of Canada (PAC).

17 James Cochran, "Recollections of Half A Century," 1864, Vertical Mss. File, pp. 17-18, PANS.

18 F.W. Vroom, *King's College: A Chronicle* (Halifax, 1941), p. 20.

19 Walter Bates, *Kingston and the Loyalists Of the "Spring Fleet" of 1783* (1889; rpt. Fredericton, 1980), p. 13.

The task facing the Loyalists was to re-establish in this "wilderness" the educational and cultural institutions left behind in America. In doing so, they accelerated the process whereby universities, libraries and other facilities were organized in colonial Maritime society. Printers, publishers, booksellers, stationers, and teachers contributed to the support and dissemination of literature, and organizations such as the Windsor Reading-Society established precedents that were followed in other communities. Consisting of approximately a dozen subscribers, the Windsor Reading-Society usually met in October or November to order periodicals for the winter months, including *Dodsley's Annual Register, The Monthly Review, The Edinburgh Magazine, Exshaw's Dublin*, and *Carey's American Museum*. Demands for the works led to a rule in 1794 which limited to a fortnight the amount of time a member might have a volume of more than 200 pages. Records maintained until 1797 reveal that as many as seven or ten volumes might be delivered to a household during the winter period.[20] Like many books in colonial society, these volumes probably had a wider audience than is discernible, for they were undoubtedly read aloud around the fireplace much in the fashion described by Sarah Ann Anderson in the Bliss Papers or by William McCulloch in his biography of the Reverend Thomas McCulloch.[21]

While family readings of poetry, essays, and periodicals may have brought amusement and literary influence to the Loyalist hearth-place, some refugees saw the advantages of extending literature into the public sphere by supporting theatrical productions in both Halifax and Saint John. Play attendance had not been a common phenomenon in the United States until the 1770s, for prior to the Revolution there had been few facilities and even fewer opportunities for companies to mount productions. The war changed all that. Leaders on each side recognized the diversion from combat offered by theatricals and the possibility for propaganda provided by productions. Whig and Tory writers both turned to satirical drama as a way of making a political point, and by the end of the hostilities there existed a dramatic repertoire and a newly-acquired taste for theatre which the Loyalists brought with them into the Maritimes.

Prior to the arrival of the Loyalists, garrison theatricals had been performed in military centres like Annapolis-Royal and Halifax. However, the Loyalist demand and taste for drama led to an increased interest in theatre and to the first performance of a play in New Brunswick, a dual production of *The Busy Body,* and *Who's the Dupe?* staged in Saint John in February 1789. The event involved the young Loyalist actors Jonathan and Stephen Sewell and the

---

20   "Journal of the Reading-Society of Windsor, Nova Scotia," Nova Scotia Historical Society, #8, MG 20, #214, pp. 2-5, 7-8, PANS.

21   Sarah Ann Anderson to Henry Bliss, 5 August 1816, Bliss Papers, MG 1, Vol. 1604, PANS; William McCulloch, *Life of Thomas McCulloch, D. D.* (Truro, 1920), p. 73.

audience included the prominent Loyalist, Colonel Edward Winslow. A theatre afficionado, the Colonel made an overnight journey down the frozen Saint John River from Kingsclear to attend the production and subsequently wrote his own play in 1795, the "Substance of the Debates of the Young Robin Hood Society."[22] A political piece lacking dramatic possibilities, this play nevertheless illustrates the way in which local themes began to be worked into the productions and prologues of regional theatre.

One such prologue, publicly delivered in the same year that Winslow's play was privately read, was "On Opening A Little Theatre in this City," a poem that buoyantly justified the Loyalists' selection of Saint John as a site for settlement and self-consciously avoided the political reasons for the city's being "rais'd" on that "dreary coast" in 1783. Printed in *The Royal Gazette and The New Brunswick Advertiser* on 20 January 1795 and still extant in handwritten form in the papers of the Loyalist Jonathan Bliss, the prologue initially assumed an argumentative position by querying the reasons for anyone's settling on the barren coast of Saint John: "What rais'd this city, on a dreary coast,/ Alternately presenting Rocks and Frost,/ Where torpid Shell-Fish hardly found a Bed/ Where Scarce a Pine durst shew a stunted Head?" The response is not the political or patriotic one that Loyalist descendants and mythologizers would project in their poetry a century later. Instead, the answer is positive and forward-looking, based on a vision of Saint John's geographical and commercial advantages ("Twas commerce — commerce smooth'd the rugged strand./ Her streets and buildings overspread the land"). Speculating on the control of "mighty Fundy's tides" through vast fleets of commerce, the poet concluded the prologue by arguing the importance of literature in refining sensibilities wearied by affliction or the pursuit of business: "Make then the muses your peculiar Care,/ 'Midst Loss, 'midst profit, still to Verse repair,/ Verse, which refines the Pleasures of Success,/ Brings Hope, and Consolation to Distress."[23]

The marriage of imagination and reason advocated in this poem reflected the emphasis on harmony and balance central to eighteenth-century thought and reiterated elsewhere in Loyalist poetry. It also points to the tempering influence literature was seen as having on the new society and to the importance it assumed as an anodyne to discouragement and regret. Jacob Bailey, Roger Viets, Jonathan Odell, Joshua Wingate Weeks, Mather Byles,

---

22 See Ann Gorman Condon, "'The Young Robin Hood Society': A Political Satire by Edward Winslow," *Acadiensis*, XV, 2 (Spring 1986), pp. 120-43.

23 "Prologue on Opening a Little Theatre at St. Johns, New Brunswick," Bliss Papers, MG 1, vol. 1610, #86, PANS. The title in the Bliss Papers substitutes "St. Johns, New Brunswick" for the more usual printed version "in This City." The poem seems to be in Bliss' handwriting and has a slightly different form of punctuation and capitalization from the published newspaper version, but it is difficult to ascertain whether Jonathan Bliss wrote the prologue or whether he copied it from the original.

Jr., and other Loyalist writers in a sense provided a "consolation to distress" for themselves and for others by continuing to write as an avocation when they left America and moved to the Maritimes. Thus, prologues like this one assumed a role as public and as important as Viets' "Annapolis-Royal" in re-affirming for Loyalists the rightness of their social vision and in reinforcing for them the importance of literature in society in refining sensibilities threatened by "Misfortune's Strokes."[24]

An even more significant contribution to the evolving cultural life of the Maritimes than reading societies and dramatic productions was the Loyalist establishment of schools, academies, and universities in the region and the introduction of a classical curriculum into the educational system. At a time when classical education was being de-emphasized in American institutions, the Loyalist founders of King's College, Windsor, encouraged and sustained a taste for poetry, language, and the humanities among scholars enrolled in the college. In the century following the founding of King's College, Windsor, in 1789, writers like Thomas Chandler Haliburton, Henry Bliss, Joseph H. Clinch, Robert Norwood, and H.A. Cody emerged from this classical curriculum, and in Fredericton, Charles G.D. Roberts, Bliss Carman, and Francis Sherman experienced a comparable training at the Loyalist-inspired University of New Brunswick. As Fred Cogswell has pointed out, the result of this non-utilitarian approach to education was that Maritime writers were prevented from committing "the barbarisms perpetrated by many frontiersmen elsewhere."[25] Schooled in translation and familiar with classical styles and verse forms, graduates perpetuated these standards of taste in their own writing and passed them on to the next generation. Although later writers knew about contemporary literary movements from their reading of current periodicals and books and from the many colonial newspapers that endeavoured to keep readers informed of developments in literary circles, a number of nineteenth-century Maritime authors chose to employ the neo-classical verse patterns and the satirical sketch form that had been favoured in the eighteenth century when Loyalist reading tastes had been shaped, and when the classical bias of Loyalist-inspired educational institutions had been established. Long after the couplet had fallen from popularity in England, it was still favoured in the Maritimes by Joseph Howe, Oliver Goldsmith, and a series of pseudonymous periodical poets of the 1820s. Similarly, the newspaper satirists of the 1820s, the "Club" members of *The Novascotian*, and Thomas Chandler Haliburton in his "Recollections of Nova Scotia" (*The Clockmaker*) all turned to the urbane, personal and ironic tone of the eighteenth-century sketch for their models. Conservatism in literary form was

---

24   *Ibid.*

25   Fred Cogswell, "Literary Activity in the Maritime Provinces, 1815-1880" in Carl Klinck, ed., *Literary History of Canada* (Toronto, 1976), I, p. 118.

therefore reinforced by the educational system and was bred by the standards of taste that Loyalist writers like Viets, Odell, Byles, and Bailey helped to establish in both their public and private work. But, while Loyalist writers softened the impact of exile on their contemporaries by encouraging a continuum in literary patterns and traditions through their work, they may also have contributed to a hardening of literary attitudes. The barbarisms of the frontier were avoided, as Cogswell has argued, but too often at the cost of originality and "the unique expression" of the writer's personality through form.[26]

A Loyalist-related literary venture that helped to define and confirm the very standards of taste about which Cogswell writes was *The Nova-Scotia Magazine and Comprehensive Review of Literature, Politics, and News*, a periodical founded by the Anglican clergyman and classical scholar, William Cochran, and produced by the Loyalist printer, John Howe of Halifax. First advertised in Saint John and Halifax on 25 May 1789 as *The Nova-Scotia Magazine, and History of Literature*, the journal promised to publish extracts from the best British magazines, review the year's new books, provide a forum for discussion on natural science, give readers the latest domestic and foreign intelligence, and encourage indigenous writing. The editor's task was to read widely and select from books and periodicals examples of the "good taste and sound sense" found in publications in Great Britain.[27] The result was to be a miscellany in the tradition of *The Gentleman's Magazine* or *The London Magazine*, although Cochran's decision to include regional and American material made the publication far more inclusive than any to be found in Great Britain.

Cochran's personal interest in education and his encouragement of literature not only shaped the editorial character of *The Nova-Scotia Magazine* but also reflected his understanding of an eclectic readership struggling to establish institutions and reinforce standards of taste in a developing area. The son of an Irish farmer and a graduate in classics from Trinity College, Dublin, Cochran had moved from New York to Nova Scotia in 1788 because of his growing disillusionment with the educational standards and social conduct of post-war America. Although not a Loyalist refugee himself, he clearly developed in his editorials and essays a vision of an agriculturally-based, ordered society sympathetic to that found in Tory circles. His editorials on the importance of farming were influential in encouraging the formation of agricultural societies, and his essays on education reinforced traditional standards in their call for well-trained

---

26 *Ibid.*, p. 119.

27 "Proposals For Publishing a Monthly Work, by the title of *The Nova-Scotia Magazine, And History of Literature*," *The Royal Gazette and New Brunswick Advertiser* (Saint John), 27 October 1789.

teachers, classical curricula, educational opportunities for the poor, and the involvement of Church and State in the educational process.[28] In the material which Cochran selected for the magazine, as well as in his own contributions, there were further revelations of the values and ideals that formed part of his social vision. Not surprisingly, the poetry that he selected from contemporary British periodicals illustrated in its late Augustan preoccupations many of the influences that had shaped and informed the reading tastes of the Loyalists before and during the war. However, it did not include satirists like Dryden, Pope, and Churchill who had provided literary precedents for the trenchant Revolutionary verse of Odell, Bailey, and Stansbury. Instead, the poetry was that of Cowper, Collins, Gray, and Wharton, the late eighteenth-century lyricists who began to relax the conventions of the couplet as they explored sentimental strains and rural themes in their work. Their unselfconscious harmonizing of the sentimental and of the traditional seemed to meet Cochran's favour as he searched out poetry and prose "to preserve and diffuse a taste for British literature,"[29] and their themes and verse forms found echo in the small body of indigenous poets who appeared in the magazine between 1789 and 1792. Eager to stimulate "young writers, among the rising generation, to try their strength, and lead them on to greater attempts,"[30] Cochran received in the contributions of "Werter," "Amintor," "J.C.," "Amicus," "Minimus" (Joshua Wingate Weeks), and "Pollio" a modest but encouraging response to the magazine's invitation for original work. Of all these, the pseudonymous "Pollio" was the most capable and the most prolific, developing in his "vanity of human wishes" theme and his pastoral motifs the tone of adaptation found elsewhere in poems like Roger Viets' "Annapolis-Royal" or Anonymous' "On Opening a Little Theatre in This City":

> Here blest with health, with peace and plenty blest,
> Should wild ambition e'er disturb my breast?
> Should discontent, or envy rack my soul,
> To see Lord Cringer in his chariot roll?
> To me more dear than all that wealth can show'r
> Sweet independence of the man in pow'r!
> While free amid my native woods to rove,
> To tend my flocks and sing the maid I love,

---

28   See "A Plan of Liberal Education For the Youth of Nova Scotia, and the Sister Provinces in North-America" which appeared in *The Nova-Scotia Magazine* under the pseudonym "W", I (August 1789), pp. 105-6; I (September 1789), pp. 199-203; and I (November 1789), pp. 364-66.

29   "To the Public," *The Nova-Scotia Magazine*, I (June 1790), n.p.

30   *Ibid.*

In falsely flatt'ring crowds I scorn to toil,
Or fawning court a titled blockhead's smile:
Below the anxious cares that plague the great,
Above the grovelling flatterer in state,
Screen'd in obscurity, from slander's sway,
In humble bliss I waste the careless day.[31]

The repetition of the word "blest" in Pollio's poem and the association of "health," "peace," and "plenty" with Nova Scotia ("Here") reinforced the forward looking tone to be found in *The Nova-Scotia Magazine* whenever the province and its sister settlements were mentioned. Given its conservative editor, William Cochran, its Loyalist printer, John Howe, and its strongly Loyalist subscription list, there would be every reason to suppose that *The Nova-Scotia Magazine* might have reflected some sense of regret about the past or some sense of bitterness about the triumph of republicanism to the south. However, the emphasis was on current international events, recent British and American publications, and social and cultural items of interest to a developing community. The temper of the journal was both positive and non-partisan, and to this end Cochran included in the magazine in February and March 1790 the full text of *The Father: or American Shandyism*, William Dunlap's conciliatory post-war American play that had been performed for the first time in the John St. Theatre in New York in the fall of 1789. The polemical dramas written during the Revolution had been followed in the United States by patriotic productions like Royall Tyler's comedy *The Contrast*, which pitted British-style effeteness against the vitality of Brother Jonathan, a stage Yankee figure designed to become a stereotype in North American literature. Dunlap's play had followed closely upon Tyler's, but differed vastly in tone by advocating friendship and the healing of old wounds between Britain and America. The reunion of the Patriot war-hero and his Tory son at the end of the play, and the marriage of the American heiress and the young British officer from Halifax, indicate Dunlap's conciliatory purpose in writing the drama. Working with the prodigal son theme so popular in literary America at the time of the Revolution,[32] Dunlap brought England back to the welcoming arms of America. Attitudes toward America had already begun to soften in many Loyalist circles, as Neil MacKinnon has pointed out,[33] and Loyalist readers of *The Nova-Scotia Magazine* certainly could not miss the open message of reconciliation

---

31   Pollio, "Rural Happiness," The Nova-Scotia Magazine, I (December 1789), p. 472.

32   Jay Fliegelman, *Prodigals and Pilgrims* (Cambridge, 1982), pp. 36-89.

33   Neil MacKinnon, "The Changing Attitudes of the Nova Scotian Loyalists towards the United States, 1783-1791" in P.A. Buckner and David Frank, eds., *The Acadiensis Reader: Atlantic Canada Before Confederation* (Fredericton, 1985), Vol. I, pp. 118-29.

expressed by Dunlap's Cartridge when he says: "I think not the worse of a soldier, or a man for being English. We are no longer enemies, your Honour."[34]

The significance which Cochran ascribed to *The Father: or American Shandyism* can be judged by his editorial note commending the work to his readers and by the fact that he reprinted no other play in his magazine during his tenure as editor. Its inclusion suggests that he may have seen his journal as playing a neutral role in his provincial constituency, especially among the Loyalist component of his readership. Circulating in a sparsely-developed and poorly-connected region as it did, *The Nova-Scotia Magazine* never had more than 300 subscribers. Yet those 300 included the colonial hierarchy in Halifax, Saint John and elsewhere; a generous proportion of Loyalist subscribers throughout the Maritimes; and the unknown listeners and borrowers of the magazine who probably swelled its readership tenfold.[35] At a time when demand for periodicals had swept England and had spread to America, Cochran clearly detected among colonial readers a taste for miscellany literature little satisfied by the colony's newspapers. Appealing to their desire to acquire a judicious blend of recent information and the best in British, American and Maritime writing, he had carefully gauged the amount of money, time, and space that could be allotted to his purpose. At four pounds a year the journal was an expensive investment for most families, but for that sum, the subscriber received 80 pages of double-column print on a monthly basis. When at least one farmer offered Cochran doggerel and potatoes instead of cash ("As cash in the country is quite out of use"), the editor accepted the arrangement with the proviso that the bluenoses be superior to the verses.[36] However, the farmer's dilemma reflected a very real problem for Cochran. While the taste and demand for the journal were real, the cash basis to support it were not. Another difficulty arose when in June 1790 Cochran was appointed to the presidency of King's College, Windsor. When he felt compelled to resign from the editor's chair because of the demands of his new position, the magazine lost the one man who had the imaginative vision, scholarly background, and eclectic interests necessary to keep it going. Thus, in spite of the best efforts of its new editor, John Howe, *The Nova-Scotia Magazine* began to lose momentum in 1791. Forced to retrench from 80 pages to 64 in January 1791, Howe gradually decreased

---

34   *The Father: or American Shandyism*, *The Nova-Scotia Magazine*, II (March 1790), p. 183. Cochran took his version of the play from *The Massachusetts Magazine*.

35   In *Sketches and Tales Illustrative of Life in the Backwoods of New Brunswick* (London, 1845), pp. 40-41, and 54, Mrs. Emily Beavan described the way periodicals were passed around in her community at Long Creek.

36   A Farmer, "Poetical Letter to the Editor of *The Nova-Scotia Magazine*," *The Nova-Scotia Magazine*, I (November 1789), p. 389. Blue potatoes were a staple in the local diet.

both the political and literary content of the periodical. By March 1792 he was forced to admit defeat, citing a small subscription list and the reluctance of subscribers to pay their bills as reasons for terminating the journal.[37]

The impact of *The Nova-Scotia Magazine* on Maritime literary life was both psychological and immediate. On a practical level, it provided an outlet for regional essayists and creative writers for a short period in the late eighteenth century and, long before such a development could otherwise have been expected, brought colonial Nova Scotia into the periodical revolution taking place in Britain and the United States. It provided a forum for discussion on topics of regional importance like education and agriculture; it provoked Maritimers into a reconsideration of their recent history by publishing extracts and letters on the events of the time; it encouraged classical education by reporting faithfully on the progress of Latin scholars at the grammar schools in Halifax and Windsor and by providing readers with translations from Pindar and Anacreon; and it kept readers informed of the latest book and periodical literature available in Britain and America. In a sense "an experiment in adult education," as D.C. Harvey has described it, the magazine reinforced the social attitudes and aesthetic tastes that the British government and the Anglican Church hoped to see firmly entrenched in Maritime society and brought a pride of accomplishment to the region early in its literary life. Although Harvey also observed that the periodical was "another muniment of that loyalist effort which could find fulfilment only in the second generation,"[38] it is significant that the next generation did not forget the example set by *The Nova-Scotia Magazine*. The editors and publishers of *The Acadian Magazine* (1826-1828) and *The British North American Magazine* (1831) both looked back to *The Nova-Scotia Magazine* as a standard against which to measure their own periodical efforts, remarking on the quality achieved by the journal in spite of the precarious economic and cultural climate in which it had tried to publish.[39] As late as 1866, the periodical was still being referred to as an important exemplar in the periodical field and as a significant contribution to the birth of Nova Scotian literary activity.[40]

The organization of publications, classical colleges, reading societies, and theatrical productions all represented Loyalist initiatives in a public sphere, and, in a sense, initiatives in a male domain. Often ignored in discussions of cultural activity because of the dearth of information available is the more

---

37 "To The Public," *The Nova-Scotia Magazine*, V (March 1792), p. 192.

38 Harvey, "The Intellectual Awakening of Nova Scotia," pp. 107, 111.

39 See "Address," *The Acadian Magazine*, I (January 1827), pp. 278-79, and "To The Public," *The British North American Magazine, and Colonial Journal*, I (February 1831), p.2.

40 James Cuppaidge Cochran, "More Recollections of Half A Century," Vertical Mss. file, p. 26, PANS.

private role played by Loyalist women in preserving and influencing standards of taste. The surviving letters of Rebecca and Eliza Byles reveal that these descendants of one of New England's most famous literary and intellectual families knew no literary time lag in Halifax as they corresponded with their Boston aunts from the 1780s to the 1830s. Their letters range easily over discussions of Francis Brooke, Sir Walter Scott, Washington Irving, and Hannah Moore. "What do you think of *Rob Roy* and all that class of novels?" Rebecca Byles was to write to her New England relatives in 1821; "they have a very popular run." "I am very much pleased with *The Sketch Book*," she adds after reading Washington Irving's recently published work. "I think it is the best American production that I have met with. The sentiments are natural and the stile chaste and elegant."[41] Elsewhere, Sarah Ann Anderson was to engage in lively analyses of fiction in her letters to Henry Bliss of Fredericton, praising the forceful language of Scott's *Guy Mannering* but criticizing the insipidness of his female characterization. "But let it always be remembered," she playfully reminds her male correspondent, "a gentleman wrote them."[42]

Rebecca Byles and Sarah Ann Anderson came from culturally sophisticated families, and their letters point to the existence of a body of women in Maritime society who had an impact on the literary tastes of the children whom they raised and taught. One of the best illustrations of the way in which this influence was exerted lies in the curriculum and the literary example set by Deborah (How) Cottnam, a resourceful teacher and poet who had been raised on Grassy Island, Nova Scotia from 1728 to 1744, but had spent the pre-revolution years in the Boston-Salem area with her husband, Captain Samuel Cottnam of the 40th Regiment. Forced to leave Salem on 29 April 1775 because of the intense local reaction against Tories, Mrs. Cottnam had retreated to Nova Scotia with the Loyalist family of George DeBlois. Faced with supporting herself, an unmarried daughter, and an invalid husband in Windsor, Mrs. Cottnam set about the task of organizing a school for gentlewomen, first in Halifax, and then in Saint John. A person of refinement and intellect, she was on intimate terms with the most influential families in both cities, and her student population included the daughters of a number of prominent Loyalists. "Mrs. Cottnam is in town at the Head of a Female Academy," Rebecca Byles wrote to her Boston aunts in 1777; "my sisters and I go to her, they to plain sewing and Reading, and I to writing, learning

---

41   Rebecca Byles to the Misses Byles, 12 March 1821, The Byles Papers, MG 1, vol. 5, #163, p. 14, PANS. Rebecca and Eliza Byles were daughters of the Loyalist and Church of England clergyman, Mather Byles, Jr. Their grandfather was the Boston clergyman, wit, and poet, Mather Byles, Sr., and their direct and collateral lineage included Cotton Mather, Increase Mather, and Richard Mather.

42   Sarah Ann Anderson to Henry Bliss, 5 August 1816, Bliss Papers, PANS.

French (Parley Vous Francois Mademoiselle) and Dancing, which employs a good Part of my time."[43] By the time she had graduated from Mrs. Cottnam's care, Rebecca Byles could confidently bandy about the name of John Locke in her letters and was proficient enough in French that she could be "imploy'd in translating a very long sermon for Doctor (John Breynton) from French into English." She was also "reading Pamela and Terences Plays in French" and was engaged "in hearing Popes Homer."[44] Boys in the colony were poorly educated, Rebecca confided to her aunts, knowing no more than how to dance and make polite conversation. "Girls," on the other hand — or seemingly the ones educated under Mrs. Cottnam — "have the best Education the place affords, and the accomplishment of their Minds is attended to as well as the adorning of their Persons." With such training behind them, argued Rebecca Byles, "In a few years I expect to see women fill the most important offices of Church and State."[45]

Approaches to women's education underwent considerable revision in America in the post-war years as Linda Kerber and Mary Beth Norton have both pointed out,[46] so that Rebecca Byles' comments on Mrs. Cottnam's influence have a strikingly contemporary ring. That Mrs. Cottnam was known to her students as a poet as well as an effective teacher becomes clear in surviving fragments of her work found in the Ward Chipman Papers and in Joseph Howe's 1845 newspaper series, "Nights With The Muses."[47] Her poem "On Being Asked What Recollection Was" illustrates her disciplined control of the couplet as a poetic vehicle, her sense of process as she brings the poem to its logical conclusion, and her ability to free herself from convention as she informally and bemusedly ends the poem on a personal rather than a formal note. The young Eliza has posed the question which gives form and title to the poem. At the completion of the exercise, there remains only human tenderness offsetting the failure of rational argument to address a child's innocent query: "Struck and Convinced, I drop the onequal [sic] task/ Nor further dare though *my Eliza ask*."[48]

Although Deborah How Cottnam set a literary example to her students and her friends, her own family best demonstrates the way in which literary

43 Rebecca Byles to the Misses Byles, November 1777, Byles Letters, MG 23, D6, PAC.

44 Rebecca Byles to her "Dear Aunt," 6 January 1779, *ibid.*

45 Rebecca Byles to her "Aunt," 24 March 1784, *ibid.*

46 See Linda K. Kerber, *Women of the Republic: Intellect and Ideology in Revolutionary America* (Chapel Hill, North Carolina, 1980), pp. 185-264, and Mary Beth Norton, *Liberty's Daughters: The Revolutionary Experience of American Women, 1750-1800* (Boston, 1980), pp. 256-94.

47 "Portia," "Birth-day Address," Ward Chipman Papers, Microfilm M-153, pp. 1-2, PAC; "Nights With The Muses," *The Novascotian* (Halifax), 16 June 1845.

48 "Nights With The Muses."

attitudes and standards of taste passed from one generation to the next. Mrs. Cottnam's work circulated privately in the Maritimes under her pseudonym "Portia," and at some point in 1845 her poems were shown to Joseph Howe. Her daughter, Martha Cottnam Tonge, was an occasional and private poet; her grandson, Cottnam Tonge, was an eloquent orator in the Nova Scotia House of Assembly; and her great-granddaughter, Griselda Tonge, was considered one of Nova Scotia's most promising young writers at the time of her death in 1825. Praised by the former Blackwood's critic, James Irving, as a fine achievement in Spenserian stanzas, Griselda Tonge's poem "To My Dear Grandmother On Her 80th Birthday" appeared in *The Acadian Recorder* in 1825, just before Griselda's death. Ostensibly a tribute to her grandmother, the poem in fact begins with a eulogium to Griselda's great-grandmother, the poetess "Portia" (Deborah How Cottnam), who had inspired a sense of literary tradition in her descendant:

> How oft from honor'd Portia's hallow'd lyre
> In tones harmonious this lov'd theme has flowed —
> Each strain, while breathing all the poet's fire,
> The feeling heart and fertile fancy showed;
> Oft times, in childhood, my young mind has glowed
> While dwelling on thy sweet descriptive lay —
> Oh, that the power had been on me bestowed
> A tribute fitting for the theme to pay! —
> With joy I'd touch each string to welcome in this day.[49]

With its appreciation of family tradition and its consciousness of literary continuity, this poem confirmed the "power" that had been "bestowed" or passed on from one generation to another. Patterns of literary and cultural taste have been little examined in Canada, nor have scholars even begun the task of assessing the influence of curricula, periodicals, libraries, reading societies, churches, and publishers on standards of public taste in this country in the eighteenth and nineteenth centuries. However, in glimpses of family literary traditions like those in the Cottnam-Tonge family, there is some insight into the effect that individual Loyalists may have had on standards of cultural taste in nineteenth-century Maritime Canada.

Described by all who knew her as "everything that (was) excellent in a Woman"[50] Deborah How Cottnam summed up her life in a letter to a friend just a few years before she died: "My morning of life was happy, but Fortune smiled deceitful; many have been the chances and changes of my pilgrimage,

---

49 "The Fount," *The Acadian Recorder* (Halifax), 5 March 1825.

50 Lois Kernaghan, "Deborah How," *Dictionary of Canadian Biography*, V (Toronto, 1983), pp. 429-30.

various the vicissitudes, poignant the afflictions."[51] The tone is familiar to anyone reading the literary works of Jacob Bailey or the personal correspondence of displaced Tories like Jonathan Sewell and Joshua Wingate Weeks. Yet, with the exception of Bailey's satires on Methodism and republicanism and Odell's later poetry on the War of 1812, the poetry, prose, and drama written by Loyalist writers in the Maritimes after the Revolution tended to be domestic, topical, and ceremonial in subject matter and forward-looking in tone. Although Ray Palmer Baker has suggested that "it is folly to argue that they [the Loyalists] made any advance in the decades after the Revolution," he does admit that to them must be given credit for "the maintenance of literary ambition."[52] The point is an important one. Thwarted in their economic and political aspirations,[53] the Loyalists nonetheless succeeded in establishing literary standards and cultural structures on which successive generations could build. The couplet form and the ironic sketch employed by both formal and vernacular writers in the eighteenth century were to remain forms of literary expression for Maritime writers well into the 1820s. Casting back to the example of their Loyalist antecedents as well as to eighteenth-century literary progenitors in Britain, Joseph Howe, Oliver Goldsmith Jr., Griselda Tonge, Thomas Chandler Haliburton, and other writers of the second or third generation could well acknowledge their practical and psychological debt to those who founded the academies, colleges, libraries, periodicals, printing establishments, and dramatic societies that had consolidated standards of taste in the region. In 1795 the writer of "On Opening A Little Theatre In This City" had advocated turning to verse as a "consolation to distress." It was also one of the "pleasures of success."

51 D. Cottnam to Nancy, 16 March 1794, Wolhaupter Papers, MC 300/ 18/ 2, p. 4, Provincial Archives of New Brunswick.

52 Baker, *A History of English-Canadian Literature*, p. 51.

53 See D.G. Bell, *Early Loyalist Saint John: The Origin of New Brunswick Politics, 1783-1786* (Fredericton, 1983) and Ann Gorman Condon, *The Envy of the American States: The Loyalist Dream for New Brunswick* (Fredericton, 1984).

James Irving:
Literature and Libel in Early Nova Scotia

In "The Intellectual Awakening of Nova Scotia," D.C. Harvey notes that the period after 1812 saw the rise of newspapers, libraries, academies, social organizations, and other institutions in Nova Scotia complementary to an emerging provincial identity. "Agriculture, fishing, lumbering and shipbuilding forged ahead," he argues, "and the minds of the young Nova Scotians were quickened both by economic rivalry and by the literature of knowledge that was written about their province."[1] The result was not only an increase in the prosperity and confidence of the colony, but also a flowering of cultural activity as "poets, essayists, journalists and historians, artists, educators, controversialists and politicians strove with or against one another to lift Nova Scotians to the level of their fellow countrymen overseas."[2]

Not least among the cultural manifestations of Nova Scotia's developing identity in the post-Napoleonic period was the emergence of literarily inclined newspapers and their concomitants — strong, regionally based writers. Agricola's 1818-21 essays on agriculture in *The Acadian Recorder* and Thomas McCulloch's 1821-23 letters on Mephibosheth Stepsure were among the most striking examples of a new literary spirit emerging in the province, but the writings of these men represented only two such contributions among many. In *The Acadian Recorder*'s satiric sketches by T.S.B. and Viator, in *The Novascotian*'s ironic letters by Patty Pry, and in Joseph Howe's rollicking newspaper presentations of "the Club" proceedings, there was ample evidence of the vitality and breadth of Nova Scotian writing throughout the decade of the 1820s. Mainly satirical in tone, it ranged over politics, agriculture, economics, education, and the vagaries of polite society. Thus, the newspaper became both a social and literary resource — everyone's political and cultural arbiter in a colonial society physically removed from the cosmopolitan mainstream of London, Edinburgh, and Boston, but increasingly conscious of its place in a wider social and cultural context.

Given the accessibility and importance of newspapers in disseminating literature in the province, it is not surprising that the Scots-born poet and critic James Irving turned to *The Acadian Recorder* as a literary outlet when he arrived in Nova Scotia in 1819. A native of southern Scotland and reputedly an Aberdeen graduate,[3] Irving seems to have had some experience

---

1 D.C. Harvey, "The Intellectual Awakening Of Nova Scotia," in G.A. Rawlyk, ed., *Historical Essays on the Atlantic Provinces* (Toronto, 1971), p. 116.

2 *Ibid.*, p. 119.

3 Israel Longworth, *A History of the County of Colchester, Nova Scotia* (Truro, 1878), II, p. 241. Irving signed himself "A.M." on official school records now lodged in the Public

in publishing with the newspaper and periodical press in his native country. Poems by "J. I—G" and "J.I." appearing in *The Dumfries and Galloway Courier* between 1812 and 1814 seem almost certainly to be by Irving, particularly if one compares a letter on Burns by "I—G" appearing in *The Courier* to two essays on "The Southern Peasantry of Scotland" by "I—G" published in *The Acadian Recorder* of Halifax in 1821. In both the author identifies himself as a staunch admirer of the peasantry amongst whom he has been raised, and in both he argues (in the words of his Dumfries article) that past association or history has enabled "the peasantry of Scotland to rise superior to the lower ranks of the community in almost every other nation under heaven, and to form their minds feelingly alive to those variations, in the economy of the natural as well as the moral world."[4] As Irving was to continue in *The Acadian Recorder,* "I have found in no quarter of Scotland, in none of England, in none of Ireland, and much less in France, or Switzerland, or Nova-Scotia, peasantry to be at all compared to them [those of the highlands of southern Scotland] in any of the qualifications of mind that exalt human nature."[5] "It will easily be perceived then," he ended this essay, "that I look upon the character of peasantry to depend almost altogether on the associations inspired by their country, and where these associations are few, or not generally interesting, in like proportion is the character."

Irving's essays on the peasantry of southern Scotland reveal how characteristic of the Romantics he was in his perception of rural life and in his association of landscape and spirituality. Hogg, Burns, Scott, and Wordsworth were always to be among the writers he most admired, partly because they represented the traditional and rural values he espoused, and partly because they had the ability to use the language "of simple feeling that Mr. Wordsworth conceives to be far more logical and philosophical in every view, than the artificial and fluctuating language of the busy world."[6] Undoubtedly this appreciation was further enhanced by Irving's association

---

Archives of Nova Scotia. The only proof of the A.M. is an irregular degree of A.M. awarded to a James Irvine by the Board of Governors of Marischal College, University of Aberdeen on 30 April 1819. See: Peter John Anderson, ed., *Fasti Academiae Mariscallanae Aberdonensis*, Vol. II (Aberdeen, 1898), p. 426. James Irving's distinctive signature does appear on the *Edinburgh University Matriculation Roll*, Vol. III (1811-29), pp. 758 (1814-16), signed Langholm and Moffat respectively as places of residence. A classmate of Irving's was William Grigor, later to be the doctor in Truro when Irving arrived there penniless in 1819.

4   I—G, "To the Editor of the Dumfries and Galloway Courier," *The Dumfries and Galloway Courier*, 28 June 1814.

5   I—G, "On the Southern Peasantry of Scotland," *The Acadian Recorder* (Halifax), 14 July 1821.

6   I—G, "Letters on the Present State of English Poetry...Letter 6, On Wordsworth," *The Acadian Recorder*, 29 July 1820.

with Edinburgh literary life in 1816-17 when James Hogg, John Wilson, and
Walter Scott were active in the city's writing circles and when the latest
production by Byron, Coleridge, or Wordsworth provoked lively discussion
in the booksellers' shops and the periodical press. That Irving was close
enough to the centre of this life to be familiar with Hogg's work in progress[7]
or to attend John Wilson's private celebrations on the anniversary of Burns[8]
is clear from his correspondence with Wordsworth now lodged in the Dove
Cottage Library in Grasmere. It is also clear from these letters that Irving kept
Wordsworth chattily informed of publishing activities and literary responses
in Edinburgh, including Irving's own involvement with the Blackwood's
group as it launched *The Edinburgh Monthly Magazine* in the spring and
summer of 1817.

William Blackwood had great ambitions for the magazine that was
eventually to bear his name, and he attempted to solicit the support of all
classes of literary men in Edinburgh in order to challenge the supremacy of
established periodicals like *The Quarterly* and *The Edinburgh Review.* Irving
seems to have been among those to whom Blackwood turned, for his name
not only appears on Blackwood's 1817 account books as a contributor,[9] but
also enters William Blackwood's correspondence in June of that year as a
reviewer deeply disturbed by the journal's attack on Wordsworth's *Letter to a
Friend of Burns.* Writing to Wordsworth on 21 June 1817, Blackwood
attempted to placate the poet by indicating that "Mr. Wilson, Mr. Gray and
Mr. Irving have expressed themselves very strongly on the subject," and by
indicating that "the last mentioned gentleman communicated to me this day
his determination to answer the obnoxious Paper in our next number."[10]
Although Irving's article does not seem to have materialized, Blackwood did
print a very positive essay on Wordsworth's work in October 1817. However,
Blackwood's conciliatory efforts did little to soothe Wordsworth's
resentment over the original Burns article, and even two years later the poet
was refusing to let *Blackwood's Magazine* "enter my doors."[11]

---

7   James Irving to William Wordsworth, 7 April 1817, Dove Cottage Library, Grasmere. I am
    indebted to the Trustees of Dove Cottage, Grasmere, England, for the permission to quote
    from Irving's letters.

8   James Irving to William Wordsworth, 1 February 1817, *ibid.*

9   Accounts Book: 1817, Blackwood Papers, Acc. 5644, H.1, p. 26, National Library of
    Scotland.

10 William Blackwood to William Wordsworth, 21 July 1817, Blackwood Papers, Acc. 5643,
    A 2, pp. 38-39, National Library of Scotland. John Wilson was in fact the author of the
    article under discussion. See "W.W. to James Irving," 22 June 1817, Letter 454, in Ernest D.
    Selincourt, ed., *The Letters of William and Dorothy Wordsworth* (2nd ed., Oxford, 1970),
    III, p. 389, n. 2.

11 "W.W. To Francis Wrangham," 19 February 1819, Letter 533, in Selincourt, ed., *Letters of
    Wordsworth,* III, p. 522.

Wordsworth's annoyance over the Burns article may have affected his relationship with *Blackwood's Magazine,* but it does not seem to have influenced his correspondence with James Irving. A letter written to Irving on 22 June 1817 was formal but civil, attacking the young reviewer's "infant publication" in uncompromising terms but clearly including Irving among Wordsworth's "friends".[12] Moreover, the poet's scepticism about the magazine's future was not original to him, for as early as 7 April 1817, Irving had expressed his concern to Wordsworth about the editorial and critical directions of the new journal with which he was associated. The editor, he had explained, "wants determination, and like all people who do not study and meditate independently, is bewildered in a maze of error and contradiction."[13] The result, Irving had noted, was that he would personally desist from having anything to do with the periodical, for "in any Work where principles are promulgated at complete variance with what I believe, I am determined not to intermeddle, unless unpurified, as they phrase it, by alteration, and this I know will never be allowed me."

It is clear, therefore, that Irving had scruples about supporting any journal that did not meet his critical criteria, and it may well have been this fastidiousness (as well as the employment opportunities afforded by a larger city) which encouraged him at the end of 1817 to follow other ambitious Scots of his generation to London. Only in London, as he was to point out years later in an essay on James Hogg, was a writer able to support himself by his pen "if he be a mere contributor."[14] Once resident in London, however, Irving was fortunate in securing a position on *The Morning Chronicle,* a newspaper edited by fellow Scot, James Perry, and renowned in Britain for its Whig politics and writers of literary ability. Appropriate as this appointment initially appeared to be, Irving's tenure on the newspaper seems to have been mysteriously short-lived and mysteriously terminated.[15] Casual references to Irving in Thomas De Quincey's letters to Wordsworth suggest Irving had some social intercourse with literary circles in the spring of 1818[16] but in March of the same year Mary Wordsworth warned her cousin, Thomas

---

12 "W.W. To James Irving," 22 June 1817, Letter 454, *ibid.,* III, p. 389.

13 James Irving to William Wordsworth, 7 April 1817, Dove Cottage Library, Grasmere.

14 I—G, "Letters on the State of English Poetry...Letter 24, On Hogg," *The Acadian Recorder,* 27 July 1822.

15 Inquiries to the newspaper library of the British Library have failed to uncover any records from *The Morning Chronicle* pertinent to Irving's dismissal. The information that he had lost his position came out in "Supreme Court, Truro: Irving vs. Ward," *The Free Press* (Halifax), 19 June 1821.

16 Thomas De Quincey to William Wordsworth, 25 March and 4 April 1818 in John E. Jordan, *De Quincey to Wordsworth: A Biography of a Relationship* (Berkeley, 1962), pp. 304, 309.

Monkhouse, not to lend money to Irving.[17] Obviously both financially and socially embarrassed, James Irving seems to have had no other recourse at this point but immigration to North America. After reputedly spending a period of time in New York City, Irving proceeded to Nova Scotia in the summer of 1819.

By the time Irving arrived in Halifax, he was forced to seek food and financial assistance from the city's North British Society. Society records for 5 August 1819 indicate that a meeting voted five pounds to a "James Erving"[18] to return to Scotland, and James Foreman, President of the Society, later remembered giving money to James Irving for bread and cheese.[19] However, by the winter of 1819-20, Irving had removed to the prosperous farming community of Truro and had sufficiently re-established his social position to become master of the grammar school at one hundred pounds per annum. Professionally settled and well situated in the home of William Dickson, an influential school trustee, he again had time to turn his attention to his criticism and writing. After unsuccessfully submitting his first work to Edmund Ward's *The Free Press* in Halifax, he joined the ranks of *The Acadian Recorder*'s writers in April of 1820. In doing so, he was placing himself in direct opposition to the conservative *Free Press* and in company with Anthony Doodledoo (S.G.W. Archibald), Agricola (John Young), Mephibosheth Stepsure (Thomas McCulloch), and other reforming spirits associated with *The Acadian Recorder*.

At the time, the two newspapers had been engaged in public warfare for well over a year. Agricola's agricultural essays published in *The Acadian Recorder* in 1818-19 had elicited considerable criticism from *The Free Press* group, and pseudonymous letters submitted to the editorial pages of the two journals had contributed to a hardening of their social and political positions. After an uneasy truce, the conflict had flared anew in the early months of 1820. This time it focused on the integrity of the Reverend Dr. William Cochran, vice-president of King's College (Windsor) and Anglican rector of Falmouth. Accused of behaving manipulatively in his conduct with the Hants County Agricultural Society, Cochran had been questioned in the pages of *The Acadian Recorder* and had been publicly identified as a secret editorial force behind Edmund Ward's *The Free Press*.[20] Also identified were four

---

17   Mary Wordsworth to Thomas Monkhouse, 3 March 1818, in Mary E. Burton, ed., *The Letters of Mary Wordsworth* (Oxford, 1958), p. 36.

18   North British Society Minute Book: 1809-39, MG 20, vol. 231, 5 August 1819, Public Archives of Nova Scotia. The name in this entry is John Erving. However, the Treasurer's book for 1815-58 (MG 20, vol. 230, August 1819) says James Erving.

19   "Supreme Court, Truro: Irving vs. Ward," *The Free Press*, 19 June 1821. All further references to this work ("SCT") appear in the text.

20   "A Friend to the Free Press," *The Acadian Recorder*, 26 February 1820. See also: *The Triumphale* (Halifax, 1820).

other King's College, Anglican members of the province's upper middle class, all of them with Loyalist connections and all of them representing an old, conservative power structure. Into this atmosphere of newspaper rivalry James Irving introduced his 25 "Letters on the Present State of English Poetry, as Exemplified in the Works of the Living Poets." As a recent immigrant and a man of letters, he may have had little sense of the history and depth of political and social animosity in Nova Scotia. Notwithstanding, he entered the fray boldly, criticizing *The Free Press* on 15 April 1820 for publishing "a most exquisite poem" by Coleridge, "whom, however, they did not, or could not name; and not only gave it a most absurd title, but, what to such a particularly correct writer would be more galling, made one of the main stanzas nonsense, by printing *friend* for *fiend.*"[21] Irving's attack on *The Free Press* did not end with this incident, for in his opening essay in the "Living Poets" series, he again accused the journal of failing to do justice to contemporary literature. In his view, the newspaper revealed its "poverty of intellect" by borrowing literary opinions from British reviews, heedlessly repeating the political biases dividing leading periodicals of the day. By contrast, he argued, his own *Recorder* essays on contemporary poets would be "candid," and would not "injure at second hand the fair fame, and moral character of any Poet, whose misfortune it is to be at the mercy of every paltry scribbler, who conceives he can comprehend either the end or the scope of his genius." In adopting this stance, he made the case that he was himself "totally free from the party spirit that at present influences, so much, the judgment of the different periodical journals of England."[22]

In spite of Irving's disclaimer, the "Letters on the Present State of English Poetry" very quickly revealed the young critic's literary, if not "party," bias. In his paper on Lord Byron on 20 May he attacked *The Free Press* for "unfeelingly" extracting *Blackwood's* "violent and ungentlemanly philippic against 'Don Juan'" and openly cited John Wilson as the author of the piece. Perhaps thinking as much of Wilson's 1817 *Edinburgh Monthly* attacks on Wordsworth's *Letter To a Friend of Burns* as of his recent comments on "Don Juan," Irving went on to castigate Wilson for knowing "how very easy it is to abuse a Brother Poet and friend in a magazine, and yet admire his poetry, and even pretend to love the man."[23] His preoccupation with this theme recurred on 3 June 1820, when he once again alluded to "the Edinburgh critic of 'Don Juan', as well as the other 'monthly magazine man' whom the Free Press has quoted, (but whose opinions are not worth

---

21 I—G, *ibid.*, 15 April 1820.

22 I—G, "Messrs. Holland & Co.," *ibid.*, 13 May 1820.

23 I—G, "Letters on the Present State of English Poetry...Letter 2, On Lord Byron," *ibid.*, 20 May 1820.

controverting)."[24] To reinforce the point, he concluded his series of letters on Byron on 17 June with yet another reference to the "borrowed criticisms" of Edmund Ward's newspaper. Noting that the extracts published by *The Free Press* questioned the morality of the poet's work, Irving challenged "the gentlemen of that firm" to explain what they found conducive to "moral well being." It was not, he argued, "by whinning *[sic]* sentimentality, nor amorous ditties set to a lover's lute, nor yet by methodistical hymns, or gospel sonnets, that poetry benefits mankind." Rather:

> Lord Byron by the reverse of all this — by holding up to our view a populous world of the human heart, (for there would be many Giaours, and Corsairs, and Laras, were the opportunity given,) and painting to us, in characters never to be erased from the mind, the inevitable consequences of abandoning ourselves, unchecked, to its natural, or acquired impulses, has done, and is doing, and will do, more real good to the world, than the editors of the Free Press would, or could do, were they to live a thousand years.[25]

In many respects, Irving's attacks on Edmund Ward's *The Free Press* can be seen as a continuation of the literary disagreements he had known in the periodical world of Great Britain. The editors of *The Acadian Recorder* implied as much when on 8 December 1821 they praised the elegance and persuasiveness of Irving's essays on the "Living Poets," at the same time expressing their own personal preference for "the poetical creed of the Edinburgh Review." I—G, as they pointed out, "has been brought up in the English school of criticism" and "obviously leans towards the latter [the poetical doctrines of the *Quarterly*]." None of this, argued *The Acadian Recorder,* detracted from the merit of Irving's essays, and should charges of "intellectual weakness or intellectual presumption" cross his path in response to his critical stands, they counselled him "to let them pass with a disdainful silence, nor lend his antagonists a borrowed greatness, by replying to them."[26]

Unfortunately, a position of "disdainful silence" seems to have been a difficult one for Irving to maintain. Possibly piqued by *The Free Press's* rejection of his early writing in Nova Scotia and certainly offended by the newspaper's critical policy, Irving did not fail to express his antipathy to the journal throughout the spring of 1820. Criticism did not sit lightly with a publisher as proud and as prickly as Edmund Ward, particularly when it emanated from *The Acadian Recorder.* By 13 June 1820, the first of *The Free Press's* reactions had appeared. Signed "Endymion" of Halifax, the letter

---

24   I—G, Letter 3, *ibid.*, 3 June 1820.

25   I—G, Letter 4, *ibid.*, 17 June 1820.

26   Editorial, *ibid.*, 8 December 1821.

masked an attack on Irving's supposed presumptuousness with an attack on Irving's critical evaluation of Swift and Byron. In his third essay on English poetry, Irving had contrasted Lord Byron's development of misanthropic villain-heroes with Dean Swift's creation of Yahoo-like characters — "paltry, dirty, filthy, mean, and abominable — like himself."[27] The emotionalism of the charge left Irving open to attack, not only for his aspersions on the reputation of Swift — "that great, that national man, that champion of virtue," as Endymion described him — but also for the "opprobrious" quality of his language. As Irving's letters were ostensibly addressed to a young student at Pictou, the Truro critic and schoolmaster appeared to Endymion not only to have abnegated critical responsibility, but also to have violated the laws of decorum:

> . . . will your young friend's vocabulary be improved by receiving the elegant expressions "paltry," "dirty," "filthy," "mean and abominable?" I must tell you that you have come too late either to increase or diminish the Draper's fame, and that the memory of the Dean of St. Patrick's, will flourish, when you — your letters — and Lord Byron's "gentlemanly scoundrels" shall have returned to their native dust. In your future hypothesis be a little less dogmatical, and examine the writings of a poetical or prosaic writer before you allow yourself to condemn him; but when condemnation becomes a disagreeable necessity let it be done in as gentlemanly a manner as possible; — nothing paltry, dirty, filthy, mean or abominable.[28]

To accuse Irving of the very faults he had attacked in Swift was to provoke him into reaction. By midsummer *The Acadian Recorder* and *The Free Press* were engaged in a literary war. Letters on the merits and demerits of Swift and Thomson flew back and forth between I—G, Endymion, Amateur, Eucharis, and Phaedon, all of them given greater immediacy by appearing so rapidly on the heels of the William Cochran affair. While still writing eloquent and lucidly argued essays in his "Living Poets" series during this period, Irving fell into emotional rhetoric in his correspondence as he defended his stand against Swift. The Dean's imagination was "eternally rioting in filth and dirt,"[29] he argued on 24 June, and a few weeks later he saw Swift's work as fit only for "the very sewers of Billingsgate."[30] The climax came on 5 August when Irving finally decided that satire would achieve what polemic had not. Couched in the form of a long verse letter addressed "To

---

27 I—G, Letter 3, *ibid.*, 3 June 1820.

28 Endymion, "To Mr. I—G," *The Free Press*, 13 June 1820.

29 I—G, "To Endymion of the Free Press," *The Acadian Recorder*, 24 June 1820.

30 *Ibid.*, 15 July 1820.

Messrs. Eucharis and Phaedon of the Free Press," the attack was a revelation of Irving's comic range and cleverness. Swift was again the target, but beneath Irving's assault on the Dean's self-serving conduct lay a criticism of Edmund Ward and *The Free Press*. Canning, Castlereagh, Hannah More, Shakespeare, and Fielding helped serve his argument as he ranged easily over the ills of "ratting," bowdlerism, and unnatural man, delivering a final philippic against hypocrisy in a footnote on those strange bedfellows, Dean Swift and the editors of *The Free Press*.

Throughout Irving's attacks on *The Free Press*, writers and their works were his focus. When he did choose to denigrate Edmund Ward and his journal, it was essentially because of his strong disagreement with Ward and his editors over the literary policy of the newspaper. Thus, it was something of a surprise and a shock to Irving and to his supporters on *The Acadian Recorder* when on 8 August Edmund Ward responded to Irving's satirical poem of a few days before by publishing a pseudonymous letter and an editorial vilifying the young critic's personal character. Purporting to be written by "A Briton" residing in Onslow just outside Truro, the letter publicly identified I — G of *The Acadian Recorder* as James Irving, a schoolmaster at Truro; deplored the "low scurrilous language" of Irving's comments on Swift; and accused Irving of being dismissed with two others from his position on *The Morning Chronicle* in London. Most damaging of all was the allegation that Irving "was the friend of Henry Hunt, Arthur Thistlewood, Major Cartwright, and other reformers," and that "he went with other Renegade Britons to their Darling United States, was with Cobbet [*sic*] a while and like him left the Union in disgust." Finally, the letter from "A Briton" portrayed Irving as arriving in Truro "in a state of raggedness and poverty," acquiring a room with William Dickson, and, since that time, saying "often in private company when the worse of Ardent Spirits, that he would Radical Nova-Scotia" ("SCT", p.193).

The letter left James Irving with no alternative but the libel courts, particularly when Edmund Ward supported the anonymous contribution with an equally damaging editorial. Ward was known in Halifax as an irascible and aggressive individual, a man quick to defend himself whether on the streets or in the courts.[31] Elements of this ready emotion entered his editorial on Irving, fanning the suspicions aroused by the letter from "A Briton" and encouraging the suggestion that Irving was too immoral a writer and too dangerous a radical to be influencing the minds of Truro's young:

> God forbid that we should possess any other sentiment than that of pity for a fellow creature in distress; but when we see the animal which has but recently been warmed into existence, turn instantly about and insult

---

31 Israel Longworth, *Life of S.G.W. Archibald* (Halifax, 1881), pp. 26-27.

the community to which he is so much indebted, by procuring the insertion of indecent and immoral writings, the better feelings of our nature yield to those of a more severe and judicial character; and we deem it our imperious duty to drag the culprit before the bar of the public. Let any man (for no modest female can peruse them without a blush) read the doggerel lines inserted in the last Recorder, and let him then declare if he can, that the author of such lines written as they expressly were to meet the public eye, is a fit and proper person "to train up a child in the way in which he should go." The laws of this country watch with a scrupulous care the means of education, and such guards are placed, as seemed to the Legislature sufficient to prevent the introduction of improper persons as teachers of our youth. Here is a man who came here a short time since in a most destitute condition, for we saw him on his arrival; and had he been the character which he described himself to be, had he held the situation in England which he says he did, nothing but a gross dereliction of duty or some flagrant offence against public order, could have thrust him forth a wanderer, upon the wide world, — a supplicant for its bounty and an object of distress; yet we find this man shortly after his arrival, employed as a schoolmaster, and openly and unblushingly applauding every infidel writer of whom he treats. The Quarter Sessions, we believe, are empowered to dismiss from his situation any man, who being employed as a schoolmaster, shall afterwards be discovered to be a person not possessing a good moral character; and if we are to judge from this man's writings, and from the circumstances under which he came to this country, we think this Irving a proper subject for its consideration. ("SCT," p. 193)

Ward's open appeal to the Court of the Quarter Sessions put Irving's teaching position in considerable jeopardy, and on 19 August 1820, *The Acadian Recorder* announced in an editorial that Irving had launched a libel suit against the publisher of *The Free Press*. The subpoena was filed on 26 May 1821,[32] and the case actually came to trial before the Supreme Court of Nova Scotia on 8 June of the same year. Throughout that period, Irving continued to submit essays on Wordsworth, Moore, and Coleridge to *The Acadian Recorder* and desisted from writing the passionate letters and satirical poetry that had initiated his difficulties with Ward. Anonymous supporters like "Colchesteriensis" and "An Inhabitant of Truro" had come to Irving's defence, however, and it seemed clear by the day of the trial that

---

32   Irving vs. Ward, RG 39, Series C, Box 164, 1821, PANS.

Ward was being accused of writing not only the editorial in *The Free Press* but also the letter of "A Briton" from Onslow.[33]

Although the trial of *Irving vs. Ward* was ostensibly one in defence of character, it quickly became obvious that it was also a trial about literary censorship and freedom of expression. The years between 1807 and 1820 had seen a "steady advance in delicacy," as Noel Perrin has pointed out in *Dr. Bowdler's Legacy,* and two of the great British journals of the day, *Blackwood's Magazine* and the *Edinburgh Review,* had disagreed vehemently over the merits of the new, expurgated edition of the *Family Shakespeare.*[34] It was in this climate of controversy over the religious and moral merits of certain writers that James Irving had undertaken to defend Lord Byron as a moral writer, had quoted indelicate passages of Jonathan Swift in discussing the dean's work, and had made favourable allusions to the writing of Voltaire. Perhaps even more damaging in the eyes of *The Free Press* and its lawyers was Irving's irreverent attack on the merits of the *Family Shakespeare* and his admission that were he to parent a daughter, he'd rather have her read unexpurgated editions of Shakespeare and Fielding than Hannah More or Sarah Trimmer:

> Poor Shakespeare! he'd scarcely now know his Othello
> In the family Edition, he's such a fine fellow: —
> But between you and I Gents, in Shakespeare I'd rather
> Have my daughter read — that is were I a father,
> As I'm thankful I am not, tho' some time or other
> I may happen to be so as well as another —
> Without altering one word, without blotting one letter,
> And I'm sure I would find her a thousand times better,
> Than should she read Hannah More half a whole life,
> Even tho' 'twere to fit her for Coelebs' wife. —
> And good Mrs. Trimmer, tho' you're such a sentry,
> That 'tis rankly impossible e'er to make entry
> To any path sin has when you're in the way,
> I had rather my daughter with Fielding should stay,
> And become his Sophia and run every risk,
> Than that e'er she should sit at your ladyship's desk.[35]

The lawyer for Edmund Ward wasted no time in appealing to the jury's sense of rectitude, reading passages of Irving's doggerel aloud and

---

33   Colchesteriensis, "Messrs. Holland & Co.," *The Acadian Recorder,* 19 August 1820.

34   Noel Perrin, *Dr. Bowdler's Legacy: A History of Expurgated Books in England and America* (New York, 1971), p. 61.

35   I—G, "To Messrs. Eucharis and Phaedon of the Free Press," *The Acadian Recorder,* 5 August 1820.

introducing words like "irreligious," "improper," and "indecent" into his commentary on the critic's writing. Irving's counsel tried to bring the evidence back to the libel action against Ward, but the defence was able to keep the question of morality and literary censorship before the jury by appealing to its sense of gentility and its fear of corruption. Arguing that the manners of the present age were more refined than were those of Shakespeare's time, Johnson of the defence "explained the nature and object of the family edition of Shakespeare" to the jury. Should the spirit of the expurgated edition be attacked without recrimination, he suggested, the "hard and honest industry" of parents who had striven to give "their sons a liberal education" would be threatened. "What would be the anguish of either of their minds, to find in the child of their hopes, an infidel and a libertine," asked Johnson:

> — how would it be encreased, if he could vindicate himself by recalling the transactions of that day, and turning their attention to the records of that Court — to their own verdict in this cause, should say: — "On your oath performing your duty to your country as a juror, you approved the principles which have made me what I am — you rewarded the man whose instructions I have followed."("SCT," p. 194)

Johnson's reference to a reward was an insidious one, but it was consistent with the defence's argument that a man of Irving's sensibility be denied the £1,000 damage demanded in the libel action. Sensitive to the direction the trial was taking, S.G.W. Archibald de-emphasized his client's claim in the summation, arguing that Irving was fighting for principle and would be satisfied with money to cover costs. The judge's intervention at this point undoubtedly had some influence on the jurors, however. Returning to Irving's alleged association with such British radicals as Henry Hunt, Arthur Thistlewood, and William Cobbett, Judge James Stewart made a legal distinction between someone's being called a Thistlewood and someone's being an acquaintance of Thistlewood. In either case, Irving was tarnished in the eyes of the public, particularly as *The Free Press* had artfully run Endymion's first retort to Irving alongside Arthur Thistlewood's trial for treason in the same issue of 13 June 1820. The proceedings of Thistlewood's trial after the Cato Street conspiracy of 1820 and the details of his execution had both been thoroughly described by *The Free Press,* and this highly sensational background to Irving's court appearance probably did little to impress the judge or jurors that he was a respectable member of society qualified to be entrusted with the care of the young. Moreover, Stewart's final charge to the jury was not designed to assist Irving's case, alleging as it did that the young critic "did write and cause to be published, immoral and obscene productions, such as no person, particularly a Schoolmaster, should give to the world" ("SCT," p.195). That the jury subsequently brought down a verdict in favour of Irving seems extraordinary in view of the prejudicial opinions entered against him by the judge, but his victory must have seemed pyrrhic indeed when he was awarded damages of only two pounds.

In the decade following the trial, James Irving continued to teach and write in the Truro area. An 1872 letter by one of his former pupils pays tribute to his scholarship, his sociability, and his knowledge of French, English, Grammar, and Geography, "for the teaching of which Irving was somewhat famed." It is characteristic of his response to his environment that his "Letters on the Present State of English Poetry" were addressed to "a young student of Pictou" (where Thomas McCulloch's famous Academy was situated), and that his nicknames for his students included "'Shad' — an abbreviation of Shadrach Howl in Stepsure's Letters published by Dr. McCulloch (incog.) about that time."[36]

However significant Irving's immediate impact as a teacher might have been on Truro in the 1820s, it is as an early critic, essayist, and defender of literary expression that he assumes importance in nineteenth-century Canadian writing. Moving to Nova Scotia at a time when the province's conservative and privileged power structure was being challenged by the forces of immigration and reform, he inevitably found himself part of that struggle when he joined the ranks of *The Acadian Recorder's* writers. *The Free Press's* response to Irving and Judge James Stewart's antipathy to his work at the trial both represent the backlash of a conservative and often Loyalist circle in the province, a force still dominated by the aesthetics and the social philosophy of the previous century. It is no surprise, then, that Irving's attacks on the literary policy of *The Free Press* antagonized its editors, or that his essays praising the imaginative powers of Byron and Wordsworth met with little sympathy from the admirers of Swift and Pope. Often printed side by side with McCulloch's satirical "Stepsure Letters," imitations of *Peter's Letters To His Kinsfolk*,[37] and Censor's provocative letters to the editor, Irving's "Letters on the Present State of English Poetry" represented yet another example of the new social and literary forces entering provincial life in the 1820s that contributed to Nova Scotia's cultural development.

Although Irving's controversy with *The Free Press* tended to obscure other public responses to his "Living Poets" series, there were those who rallied to

---

36   D. McCurdy to Jane, 2 March 1872, Longworth Manuscripts (Scrapbook), 1-200, Mount Allison University Archives.

37   John Gibson Lockhart published *Peter's Letters to his Kinsfolk* in 1819. A series of ironic sketches about Scottish society, they were extremely popular. *The Acadian Recorder* published a local series called "Paul's Letters to his Kinsfolk," 18 August to 29 December 1821. While vastly different in subject matter from McCulloch's "Stepsure Letters," they nonetheless complemented *The Recorder's* publication of comic sketches.

Irving's defence before and after the trial to express their appreciation for the polish and persuasiveness of his essays. "Byron, Coleridge, Moore, etc. were wholly unknown to many in this province, until you announced them as poetical characters," wrote "W." of Horton Corner in November 1821,[38] and his sentiments were repeated by a young man from Pictou, "C.C." of Parrsborough, and the Hollands of *The Acadian Recorder*.[39] I do not speak rashly," added "Willoverthewater" in December of 1821, "when I say they are letters of talent;...nor do I flatter when I say that they, in many instances, attain the highest pitch of pure criticism — criticism that should direct if not lead the public taste: in them the mien, manner, and thought, have been duly studied, deeply considered, and finely communicated."[40]

Such encomiums encouraged Irving to keep writing in both a creative and a critical vein, and throughout the 1820s he continued to contribute poetry, narratives, and essays to *The Acadian Recorder* and *The Acadian Magazine*. However, he was not again to involve himself in literary controversy, maintaining instead that "disdainful silence" *The Acadian Recorder* had once advised him to assume when facing literary detractors. That he maintained contact with other Nova Scotian writers, however, is illustrated by his support of Windsor poetess, Griselda Tonge, in 1825;[41] by "Peter's" correspondence in *The Acadian Recorder* in 1827;[42] and by an 1829 reference in the "Club" papers to the doctor's spending a night in Truro with "Jamie Irving, the profoundest of critics and the very best of good fellows."[43]

Years later, Joseph Howe was to suggest in *The Novascotian* that dissipation eventually destroyed Irving's health and affected his ability to write.[44] Regrettable as this might be, there is no denying the contribution Irving made to the intellectual development of Nova Scotia in the 1820s through the contemporaneity of his criticism, the quality of his writing, and the courage of his literary convictions. He had argued before the Truro literary society in 1821 that "as the soil so is the plant, and where the soil presents nothing but opposing barriers, culture can do little more, if it can do

---

38 W., "To I—G of Colchester," *The Acadian Recorder*, 10 November 1821.

39 See "To I—G," *ibid.*, 11 May 1822; C.C. of Parrsborough, "To I—G of Colchester," *ibid.*, 24 November 1821; "To Correspondents" and Editorial, *ibid.*, 2 June and 8 December 1821.

40 Willoverthewater, "To 'W' in the Recorder of 10th ult. respecting his address to I—G," *ibid.*, 8 December 1821.

41 I—G, "The Fount," *ibid.*, 5 March 1825.

42 Peter, "For the Recorder," *The Acadian Recorder*, 8 December 1827. For further information on Irving's relationship to *The Acadian Magazine* and the Peter correspondence, see Gwendolyn Davies, "A Literary Study of Selected Periodicals From Maritime Canada: 1789-1872," (Ph.D. thesis, York University, 1979), pp. 84-88.

43 "The Club," *The Novascotian*, 4 June 1829, p. 178.

44 "Nights With The Muses. No. 4," *ibid.*, 16 June 1845.

that, but prevent actual deterioration."[45] In his writing and in his critical stand, James Irving did much to break down the "opposing barriers" and to prepare the soil in which the intellectual flowering of Nova Scotia could take place.

---

45   I—G, "On the Southern Peasantry of Scotland," *The Acadian Recorder*, 14 July 1821.

Penetrating into Scott's Field:
The Covenanting Fiction of Thomas McCulloch

On 15 December 1828, publisher William Blackwood wrote apologetically to Dr. John Mitchell of Glasgow rejecting the novels of the Reverend Thomas McCulloch of Pictou, Nova Scotia. "I have used you very ill," began Blackwood, "and I have no apology to offer for my having so long delayed writing you, except the difficulty I have felt, and still feel in explaining to you the impressions which your friend Dr. McCulloch's MSS. have made upon me." The novels were funny, noted Blackwood. They were rich in detail. They reflected the presence of an "informing genius." But they were also coarse, localized, and, in the case of the romance, *Auld Eppie's Tales*, "penetrating, as it were, into Scott's field." As such, the latter had to be done with "exquisite skill," noted Blackwood, and under no circumstances, could be considered vulgar. "The humour and satire have all the pungency and originality of Swift," Blackwood continued in a subsequent letter, "with I am sorry to say too much of his broad and coarse colouring. Taste in these things has now a days got even more refined, and what was fit for the tea table in the days of Queen Anne would hardly be tolerated now in the servant's hall."[1]

To the Reverend Thomas McCulloch of Pictou, these were inflammatory and fighting words. Born in Ferenze, Renfrewshire, in 1776; educated for medicine at Glasgow; prepared for the Secessionist Church under Professor Archibald Bruce at Whitburn; ordained at Stewarton in 1799; called to the parish of Pictou, Nova Scotia, in 1803; and founder of Pictou Academy in 1816, the Reverend Thomas McCulloch was hardly the sort of man to whom adjectives like "course," "pungent," and "broad" would lightly be applied. The author of *Popery Condemned By Scripture and The Fathers* (1808), *The Prosperity of the Church In Troublous Times* (1814), and *Words of Peace* (1817), among other theological treatises, he had earned a reputation for activism since immigrating to Nova Scotia but hardly one for bawdry. "My novels I see will not do," he responded to Mitchell when news of Blackwood's rejection arrived in Pictou, "There is too much dirt in them...Now dirty as Bl. thinks my novels I judge them purity itself compared with his magazine [*Blackwood's Magazine*]. And it would be a subject of serious consideration with me whether I ought to write for a publication whose tendency is so irreligious." "Pray have the goodness to send for the manuscripts without waiting for his ultimatum seal them up with my name upon them and lay them past," he continued in a subsequent letter; "I do not care two pence about my publication. About writing for his magazine I have

---

1   William Blackwood to John Mitchell, 15 December 1828, Blackwoods Letter-books, Acc. 5643/B8, National Library of Scotland [N.L.S.].

only to say that I regard it as a very bad book and except in the expectation of helping to render its texture more moral I do not do it."[2]

The result of Blackwood's rejection and of McCulloch's ire was that the Pictou author never again submitted a manuscript to the Edinburgh publisher, but behind the confrontation of two seemingly strong personalities lay a context of religious tradition in one case and of publishing acumen in the other that probably guaranteed a clash of wills. By 1828, Blackwood held an unassailable reputation in the publishing world. But the daring young bookseller who had flouted convention in 1817 with the Chaldee Manuscript and had supported the satire and irreverence of the *Noctes Ambrosianae* was, by the late 1820s, also a shrewd enough businessman to be concerned about a soft economic climate for publishing. For that reason, as Blackwood's letters to Mitchell indicate, the publisher was particularly sensitive to the public's shift toward gentility in recent years, and his bowdlerization of some of John Galt's manuscripts[3] had already set the stage for his rejection of Thomas McCulloch on the grounds of indelicacy and Swiftian humour.

Compounding Blackwood's concern about the saleability of at least one of McCulloch's manuscripts, *Auld Eppie's Tales*, was its "penetration," as he put it, into "Scott's field." In a letter to Mitchell written from Pictou on 16 January 1828, McCulloch had made it clear that his motivation in beginning the novel had been, in part, a response to Mitchell's encouragement and, in part, a reaction to Walter Scott's *Tales of My Landlord*:

> Mindful of our friendship in Edinburgh and elsewhere I write this to inform you that I am complying with your wish like a slave at the oar. In a few weeks I shall have the first volume finished. Of my counter-acting story I shall leave you to judge when you read it. Though it may not come within sight of the Tales of My Landlord still I hope it will be read and amuse. I have begun with the days of popery and intend to carry on through three volumes without meddling with anything but popery and the progress of Lollardism in the west of Scotland not forgetting a due quantity of witches kelpies and other gods whom our fathers worshipped.[4]

By 24 June 1828, McCulloch was well advanced on his project, making it clear in a letter to James Mitchell, Dr. John Mitchell's son, that it was Scott's depiction of the Covenanters in *Old Mortality* (1816) that spurred him on.

---

2   Thomas McCulloch to James Mitchell, 18 May and 3 December 1829, Thomas McCulloch Papers, MG 1, Vol. 553, Nos. 39 and 46, PANS.

3   P.H. Scott, *John Galt* (Edinburgh, 1985), pp. 72-73.

4   Thomas McCulloch to James Mitchell, 16 January 1828, Thomas McCulloch Papers, MG1, Vol. 553, No. 28, PANS.

While McCulloch did not explain his specific grievances against *Old Mortality*, it is likely that he, like other Covenanter sympathizers, was offended by Scott's portrayal of them as rigid and extreme. "Like Burns, Scott disapproved of much about the Covenanters," notes David Stevenson, "but nonetheless he accepted that there were elements of value and interest in their legacy." While Scott made an effort to understand "their psychology and motivation" in *Old Mortality*, argues Stevenson, "and acknowleged their struggle as contributing to the coming of the 'Glorious Revolution' of 1688-89,"[5] it is clear in McCulloch's letter to Mitchell in June 1828 that McCulloch found Scott's interpretation of the Scotch Worthies anything but sympathetic:

> By your advice I have undertaken a business for which I have strong suspicion that Sir Walter Scott going before me I am ill qualified and which were it not a sort of vindication of our ancestors and their support of...religious truth I would account not very clerical.[6]

Six months later as he sent off a new title page and the remaining portion of Volume 3 to Mitchell, he could only reiterate that, as amusing as he tried to make the work for a general readership, a compelling motivation for his writing it had been his desire to "procure additional regard for Scotch worthies and their general principles." If he succeeded in so doing, he added, then the writing of the novel "would be well spent labour."[7]

Blackwood's preliminary reading of Volumes 1, 2, and parts of Volume 3 of *Auld Eppie's Tales* clearly alerted him to the motivation informing McCulloch's manuscript. While praising the romance to John Mitchell in his letter of 15 December 1828, Blackwood not only rejected the "coarseness" of "several of the sketches" but also queried whether McCulloch "has rather been urged on from a wish to give a different position from what Scott has drawn in his novels and tales." "That a very different picture from Scott's ought to be given," noted Blackwood, "neither you nor I will have any doubt, but it is always a doubtful affair the writing a work of fiction principally for a particular purpose." "Penetrating as it were into Scott's field," he added, "a work of this kind requires to be done with exquisite skill..."[8]

---

5   David Stevenson, *The Covenanters. The National Covenant and Scotland* (Edinburgh, 1988), p. 78.

6   Thomas McCulloch to James Mitchell, 24 June 1828, Thomas McCulloch Papers, MG1, Vol. 553, No. 33, PANS.

7   Thomas McCulloch to James Mitchell, 29 December 1828, Thomas McCulloch Papers, MG1, Vol. 553, No. 37, PANS.

8   William Blackwood to John Mitchell, 15 December 1828.

That he had touched a nerve with McCulloch is clear in the latter's response to James Mitchell on 18 May 1829. "I have never intended to be an imitation of Sir Walter," he notes; "I have neither his knowledge nor his talents. But on the other hand I conceived that the kind of information and humour which I possess would have enabled me to vindicate where he has misrepresented and to render contemptible and ludicrous what he has laboured to dignify." "As for the Lollards (a reference to *Auld Eppie's Tales*)," he adds in a subsequent letter, "I wished him (Blackwood) to get the offer of it on account of the kindness which he showed me."[9] But not all Blackwood's kindness in entertaining McCulloch on a visit to Edinburgh in 1826 or in his donating books to Pictou Academy could ever assuage what McCulloch now felt to be a slight to his reputation and a reluctance to set the record straight on the Covenanters. Blackwood's rejection of *Auld Eppie's Tales* struck at everything that McCulloch represented. On a personal level, he was descended, as his son notes, "from the McCullochs...of Galloway, and claimed kinship with Covenanters." "A tradition in the family," adds William McCulloch, "credits an ancestor with the honour of having fought at the Battle of Bothwell Bridge."[10] On a spiritual and professional level, McCulloch was a Secessionist Presbyterian clergyman, one of that band of Presbyterians who at the formation of the new Secession Church in 1737 asserted, as David Stevenson has pointed out, "the perpetual obligation on Scotland of the National Covenant" of 1581 and 1636 and "the Solemn League and Covenant" of 1643, "and acceptance of the Covenants" as "a condition for admission to communion." Unquestionably, then, the Covenanting tradition of Scotland informed every dimension of McCulloch's life, including the increasing association of the Covenants in the late eighteenth and early nineteenth centuries with populist agitation for democratic reform and justice. Both of these causes were ones that McCulloch was to champion in his theological, educational, and fictional writings from Pictou throughout the 1820s and 1830s.[11]

Little could William Blackwood understand, therefore, the depth of McCulloch's obsession with rectifying what he saw as the unsympathetic attitude to the Covenanters represented by Scott. Interestingly, neither Blackwood nor McCulloch makes reference to James Hogg's *The Brownie of Bodsbeck* (1818) or John Galt's *Ringhan Gilhaize, or, The Covenanters* (1823), the latter presumably a response to Scott's novel as much as was McCulloch's.[12] While McCulloch may have been unaware of the Hogg and

---

9   Thomas McCulloch to James Mitchell, 18 May and 4 September 1829, Thomas McCulloch Papers, MG1, Vol. 553, Nos. 39 and 43, PANS.

10 William McCulloch, *The Life of Thomas McCulloch, D.D.* (Truro, 1920), p. 7.

11 Stevenson, *The Covenanters*, p. 73, 75-76.

12 *Ibid.*, pp. 78-79.

Galt novels, Blackwood was undoubtedly conscious of the relative lack of attention that these two Covenanting works had received in the face of Scott's more controversial and dynamic work. Faced during a publishing recession with a massive three-volume manuscript by an anonymous Pictou, Nova Scotia, novelist, Blackwood may therefore have felt that the better part of common sense lay with caution.

Blackwood's rejection of *Auld Eppie's Tales* discouraged McCulloch temporarily but could not dim his determination to earn for the Covenanters and their self-sacrificing principles the fictional admiration that he felt they deserved. As early as his satirical Mephibosheth Stepsure letters published in the *Acadian Recorder* of Halifax from 1821-23, McCulloch had begun to give imaginative voice to the Scottish descendants of the Covenanting tradition. Usually commended for their comic exposé of the manners and mores of small town Nova Scotia in the post-Napoleonic period, the Mephibosheth Stepsure letters also present as one of their satirical norms the idiosyncratic figure of Saunders (Alexander) Scantocreesh, a feisty, rigid, and totally original Scot whose hard work, God-fearing principles, and economical lifestyle have brought him prosperity. Scantocreesh is in many respects a reincarnation of the spirit of the Covenanters. Faithful to principles of moral rectitude, he calls upon the Bible and the Confession of Faith when his daughters want to go to dancing school, invokes the memory of the Scotch Worthies, Claverhouse, and the Highland Host for those who do not live virtuously, and prescribes terrible punishments (eating her own tongue to the root) for deviants from the true path.[13] While McCulloch pokes fun at Scantocreesh's rigidity, he leaves no doubt of his admiration for Saunders's faith and sincerity.

These qualities are given more emphasis in Book II of the Stepsure letters when the story of "William" begins with the example of William's great-grandfather, a martyred Covenanter who "had been taken, to cement" his principles "with his blood in the Grass Market of Edinburgh, that noble structure of civil and religious privilege which is the glory of Scotland."[14] In the contemporary example of William's saintly father, and in the intertwining tendrils of ivy planted by that "worthy martyr," his great-grandfather,[15] there are symbols at the beginning of the story of how far William is to fall from the ideal of his Covenanting heritage when he immigrates to Halifax to make his fortune. In the matched tale of "Melville," published with "William" in 1826 as *Colonial Gleanings: William and Melville*, McCulloch continued to develop the Covenanting tradition as a

---

13 Thomas McCulloch, *The Mephibosheth Stepsure Letters*, ed. Gwendolyn Davies (Ottawa, 1990), pp. 47, 58, 170.

14 *Ibid.*, p. 233.

15 *Ibid.*, p. 68.

spiritual and cultural norm against which the success or failure of his protagonist is measured. It is Melville's great-grandfather who has hunted down William's great-grandfather, has caused his subsequent torture "till the blood spurted from the legs of the prisoner, and the marrow oozed from his bones," and has generated his death in the Grass Market. Infamy and decline have dogged Melville's family since, until at the beginning of the story Melville dwells in relative penury in Southern Scotland amongst descendants of the Cameronians, God-fearing members of the Reformed Presbytery who "profess to be the successors of that suffering remnant, who, in times of persecution and martyrdom, loved not their lives unto the death."[16] More dramatically than in "William," McCulloch develops two moral exemplars in "Melville" as foils to the erring protagonist. One, at the beginning of the story, is the weaver Andrew Welwood, a Cameronian/Reformed Presbyterian who in the tradition of his Covenanting ancestors "was an invincible polemic; a violent opposer of what he conceived to be Erastianism, latitudinarianism, and sectarianism of every description; and a settled believer, that every denomination of Christians, except his own, was involved in a course of defection from the purity attained by the Church of Scotland in her reforming times. For that cloud of witnesses who, in the season of persecution, had maintained the truth with testimony of their blood, he cherished a deep veneration."[17] The second moral exemplar developed in "Melville" is the Reverend James McGregor of Pictou, the Secessionist Presbyterian clergyman who had preceded McCulloch in immigrating to the Pictou region and who was always to be affectionately known by him as "father." In his piety, simplicity, dedication to principle, and self-sacrifice, McGregor represented to McCulloch the conduct and righteousness that he associated with his Covenanting ancestors. In celebrating his colleague in "Melville" in 1826 and in the Morton stories of 1833, McCulloch was engaged in the process of "vindicating our ancestors," that mission that he described to Mitchell in 1828 as his motivation for writing *Auld Eppie's Tales*. The Mephibosheth Stepsure letters, the William story, the Melville story, and the later Morton Stories are therefore central to an understanding of *Auld Eppie's Tales*, for they reveal McCulloch's developing commitment in the 1820s and 1830s to articulating in his fiction both Scotland's debt to the Covenanters and Nova Scotia's link to a Scottish Secessionist past.

Auld Eppie's Tales was never published after Blackwood's rejection of it, although McCulloch did submit it to a London bookseller in 1831.[18] It was

---

16   [Thomas McCulloch], *Colonial Gleanings: William and Melville* (Edinburgh, 1826), pp. 74-75, 68.

17   *Ibid.*, p. 71.

18   J. Blanchard to Thomas McCulloch, 30 September 1831, Thomas McCulloch Papers, MG 1, Vol. 553, No. 105, PANS.

eventually returned to the McCulloch family in manuscript form and since the 1930s has been lodged in the Public Archives of Nova Scotia in an unbound and semi-organized form. In 1981, Honours student Heather MacFadgen of Mount Allison University attempted to impose some order on the novel and made a 491-page typescript of it. However, the existence of other manuscript segments of the romance makes a definitive reconstruction somewhat difficult. Narrated retrospectively by a speaker who revisits his boyhood Renfrewshire and repeats one of the tales found in Auld Eppie's trunk, the novel strikes two notes: first, the loss of an old way of life in Renfrewshire as "cotton mills," "bleach-fields," "printfields," and an "intruding horde of eager faced, bustling beings" invade the landscape;[19] and, secondly, the ingenuity and courage of a tenant farmer, Jock O'Killoch, and some of the local lairds on the Levern River in withstanding the authority of Church and State during the reign of James III. The anti-establishment nature of the novel conforms well to McCulloch's celebration of Covenanting courage and martyrdom in his other writing, and the "Reform message grows," as Anne Wood has pointed out in "The Significance of Calvinism in The Educational Vision of Thomas McCulloch," "as the tale continues." When a stranger recites before the persecuted and increasingly admirable protagonist, Jock O'Killoch, the message "that the scriptures should be the rule of faith, should be written in the vernacular in order to be read by all people, and that the conduct of clergy should be guided by sound doctrine,"[20] the sympathetic foundation of Covenanting principles on which McCulloch hoped to refute Scott's depiction of the early Covenanters in *Old Mortality* becomes more obvious.[21]

In spite of his reverses, McCulloch did not abandon his fiction-writing after *Auld Eppie's Tales*. By 3 December 1829 he was rather combatively indicating to Mitchell that his new work might "make Blackwood wish to be my publisher."[22] He would never again give Blackwood that opportunity, however, and when on 9 November and 29 December 1833 he wrote to Mitchell about his new tale on the Reverend James McGregor, it was to Oliphant's of Edinburgh that he was planning to submit it. Here, as in "Melville," McCulloch placed McGregor in a setting deliberately evocative of the killing times. As Robert Morton, the protagonist, attends one of McGregor's services in a forest clearing near Pictou, "his musings were interrupted by the appearance of a soldier who with military step moved

19 [Thomas McCulloch], *Auld Eppie's Tales*, ed. Heather MacFadgen, ts, Honours thesis, Mount Allison University, 1981, p. 6.

20 B. Anne Wood, "The Significance of Calvinism in the Educational Vision of Thomas McCulloch," *Vitae Scholasticae*, Vol. 4, Nos. 1 & 2 (Spring/Fall 1985), p. 19.

21 *Ibid.*

22 Thomas McCulloch to James Mitchell, 3 December 1829, Thomas McCulloch Papers, Vol. 553, No. 47, PANS.

slowly along the fronting elevation. It was a Covenanter's scene and reminded Morton of those times when the intrusions of cruelty interrupted the outpourings of mercy. But there was neither the sound of the trumpet nor the alarm of war: there was no Claverhouse to stain the beauty of holiness with the blood of the saints."[23] Nonetheless, Claverhouse was an active and bloody presence in the last of McCulloch's Covenanting fictions, a 400-page novel entitled "The Days of the Covenant" that he planned to submit to Oliphant in 1834. Partly focusing on Archbishop Sharp in the seventeenth century and on what McCulloch described as "our afflicted fathers,"[24] the novel survives in fragmented form in the Public Archives of Nova Scotia. Seemingly more vivid in parts than *Auld Eppie's Tales*, it may nonetheless have suffered the same rejection as the earlier Covenanting novel, for on 18 July 1834, McCulloch wrote rather dispiritedly to Mitchell in Glasgow: "Have the goodness to say to my friend that I wish no more publishing applications. I have not talents bearing pace with the judgment of the public and *sutor ne ultra crepidam* is a sensible maxim. Necessity does not now force me to write."[25] In fact, necessity of a different sort was confronting McCulloch's authorship. If the reading public of the 1820s had possibly become sated with Covenanting stories, there was even less likelihood of McCulloch's having success with the theme in 1834. His "Stepsure" letters may, as Northrop Frye has suggested, have marked the founding of genuine Canadian humour.[26] But as a writer of Covenanting stories, McCulloch was always to remain Canada's "Great Unknown."[27]

23   [Thomas McCulloch], Thomas McCulloch Papers, Vol. 555, No. 79, PANS.

24   Thomas McCulloch to Mitchell, 29 December 1833, Thomas McCulloch Papers, Vol. 553, No. 59, PANS.

25   Thomas McCulloch to John Mitchell, 18 July 1834, Thomas McCulloch Papers, Vol. 553, No. 60, PANS.

26   H. Northrop Frye, "Introduction," in Thomas McCulloch, *The Stepsure Letters* (Toronto, 1960), p. ix.

27   This name was given by James Ballantyne to the author of the "Waverley" novels, although, from the beginning, many suspected that Walter Scott was indeed the "Great Unknown." See: William A. Wheeler, *An Explanatory and Pronouncing Dictionary of the Noted Names of Fiction* (Boston, 1883), p. 158.

"Dearer Than His Dog":
Literary Women in Pre-Confederation Nova Scotia

In past years scholars like Wilfrid Eggleston and Alfred Bailey have tended to approach nineteenth-century Maritime literature by adopting a peaks-and-valleys thesis, arguing that original figures like Thomas Chandler Haliburton, Joseph Howe, Charles G.D. Roberts, and Bliss Carman loomed large on a literary horizon otherwise characterized by works of merely regional or historical interest.[1] For Eggleston, the "golden age" of literature in the Maritimes emerged in the 1820s and 1830s when the political and intellectual fervour of society generated works like Oliver Goldsmith, Jr.'s *The Rising Village* (1825) or Thomas Chandler Haliburton's "Recollections of Nova Scotia" (1835). However, after the appearance of Sam Slick in 1835 Eggleston sees "the mountain peaks" falling away "to very modest foothills," and it is only with the post-Confederation writers, Roberts and Carman, that he again senses the excitement of true literary worth.[2]

What is ignored by this Canadian version of the Great Tradition thesis is the continuum and momentum of Maritime literary activity throughout the eighteenth and nineteenth centuries. While no one can argue with the excitement of a period that produced the letters of Mephibosheth Stepsure, *The Rising Village, The Novascotian's* "Club" series, the "Western" and "Eastern Rambles," and *The Clockmaker,* Eggleston's "golden age" thesis ignores the on-going contribution of countless newspaper and periodical authors who helped shape Maritime literary development.[3] Significant among these were the literary women who transcended the educational, economic, and geographical limitations of colonial society to achieve the publication of their work and to conduct professional literary and editorial careers. Rarely in a position to cultivate the London, Edinburgh, and Boston publishing houses that ensured visibility and distribution to such male counterparts as Thomas

---

1   See Wilfrid Eggleston, *The Frontier and Canadian Letters* (Toronto, 1957), pp. 66-67, 101-12; and Alfred Bailey, "Creative Moments in the Culture of the Maritime Provinces" in G.A. Rawlyk, ed., *Historical Essays on the Atlantic Provinces* (Toronto, 1967), pp. 229-31.

2   Eggleston, *The Frontier and Canadian Letters*, p. 67.

3   Thomas McCulloch's untitled letters of Mephibosheth Stepsure appeared in *The Acadian Recorder* (Halifax) from 22 December 1821 to 29 March 1823. *The Rising Village* by Oliver Goldsmith, Jr., was published by Sharp of London in 1825. The "Club" Papers of Joseph Howe and company (8 May 1828-12 October 1831), the "Western Rambles" and "Eastern Rambles" of Joseph Howe (23 July- 9 October 1828; 17 December 1829-19 October 1831) and the "Recollections of Nova Scotia" of Thomas Chandler Haliburton (began appearing 24 September 1835; completed for book publication as *The Clockmaker: Or, The Sayings and Doings of Samuel Slick of Slickville* in 1836) — all appeared in *The Novascotian* (Halifax), edited by Joseph Howe.

McCulloch, Thomas Chandler Haliburton, Bliss Carman, and Charles G.D. Roberts, these provincial women writers were often destined to disappear from the eye of posterity by the very ephemerality of the periodicals and private editions in which they published. As a result, their writing has rarely been anthologized, analyzed, or consciously preserved, and only a study of surviving newspapers, literary journals, private editions, commonplace books, and family papers in the Maritimes and New England can reveal something of the character and range of the imaginative writing done by these women in the Maritimes from 1749 to Confederation.

Collections of family letters such as the Byles and Bliss correspondence in the Public Archives of Nova Scotia make it clear that a core of educated women of literary sensibility existed in the Maritimes from the 1700s onwards.[4] Because of the eighteenth and early nineteenth-century convention of employing pseudonyms to disguise the authorship of poems and sketches submitted to the periodical press, it is difficult to estimate the number of literarily inclined women who were published in the Maritimes before 1825. What is clear, however, is that those seeking financial support could ill afford to rely on fledgling colonial presses or on publication by subscription to supply their needs, and writing was, therefore, very much an avocation, not a vocation, for women in the Maritimes until the mid-nineteenth century.[5] After that period, women began to assume some leadership in publishing and editing, and a number of regional women authors began to establish the links with British and American publishing houses that gave them a paid and professional status.

One early Maritime poet of ability who had to subordinate her literary interests to earning a living was Deborah (How) Cottnam (1728-1806), a woman of strong character and intellect who supported her daughter and herself after 1774 by conducting schools in Salem, Halifax, and Saint John respectively. Raised on Grassy Island, Nova Scotia, Deborah Cottnam received an atypical education for a woman of her time. Her father, Edward How, was a merchant and civilian official of "respectable" background who

---

4   The Byles Letters include the correspondence of Rebecca and Eliza Byles to their aunts in Boston from the 1770s (when the Byles daughters came to Halifax as Loyalists) until 1829. The Bliss Letters include the lively correspondence of Sarah Ann (Anderson) Bliss from 1816 to the 1840s. Both collections are housed at the Public Archives of Nova Scotia. The Byles Letters can be found in MG 1, vol. 163, and the Bliss Letters in MG 1, vols. 1595-1613.

5   Fredericton-born novelist Julia Catherine Beckwith Hart published *St. Ursula's Convent, or The Nun of Canada* by subscription in 1824 (her preface lists sponsors from Great Britain, the Maritimes, Upper Canada, and the United States). However, there is no evidence that publishing by subscription was a common practice among Maritime women writers of this period.

spoke fluent French and Micmac.[6] While he probably directed her early schooling, she later received tuition from Samuel Cottnam, an Irish-born officer in the 40th Regiment at Canso who had been well educated in England.[7] The result was that she received an academic grounding unusual for women in Nova Scotia in the 1730s and 1740s, and it was this education that stood her in good stead when political and personal events during the years of the American Revolution threw her upon her own resources. Opening a female academy in Salem, Massachusetts in 1774, in Halifax in 1777, and in Saint John in 1786, Deborah Cottnam endeavoured to train the minds of her students in the mathematical, language, and writing skills that would prepare them for a changing society. Phrases such as "with propriety," "correctness...attended to," and "as far as the rules of practice" punctuate her advertisements for her Saint John boarding school and suggest that discipline as well as the acquisition of knowledge was part of her teaching philosophy.[8] Rebecca Byles, one of her students and a member of the scholarly Cotton Mather-Mather Byles family, reinforced this impression in a series of letters she wrote her aunt in Boston after she had completed her education in Deborah Cottnam's Halifax academy.[9] Describing her activities in the months following her graduation in 1779, she noted that she had been "employed in translating a very long Sermon for Doctor Breynton, from French into English," "in reading *Pamela* and Terence's plays in French," and "in hearing Pope's *Homer*."[10] The situation of education in the colony, Rebecca observed

---

6   Martha Tonge, "Martha Tonge (Mrs. Winckworth Tonge) to Lieut. R.U. Howe (A.D.C. to Sir Howard Douglas) 81st Regiment, dated at Windsor, 1 December 1828," in *Report of the Board of Trustees of the Public Archives of Nova Scotia for the Year 1961* (Halifax, 1962), Appendix C, p. 21.

7   Tonge, *Report*, pp. 21-22. Deborah How and Samuel Cottnam married in 1743.

8   In the advertisement for Deborah Cottnam's Salem boarding school for "young ladies," she mentions the "genteel company" to which students would be introduced in her "pleasant and commodious" house near the Episcopal Church (see *Essex Gazette* [Salem], 19 July 1774). Her Saint John advertisement places more stress on her academic curriculum, although she does promise to pay attention to the "morals and manners" of her charges at the end of her advertisement. (See *The Nova Scotia Gazette and The Weekly Chronicle* [Halifax], 6 January 1789). Tuition and board cost 30 pounds per annum at her Saint John establishment, a large sum for women's education at the time.

9   Rebecca Byles was the daughter of the Reverend Mather Byles, Jr., D.D., a graduate of Harvard and the rector of Old North (Christ Church), Boston, from 1768-75. At the time of the American Revolution, he remained loyal to the Crown and removed to Halifax. He eventually became rector of Trinity Church, Saint John. Mather Byles, Jr., was the son of the well-known Boston wit, poet, and clergyman, Mather Byles. His grandfather was Cotton Mather, and his great-grandfather was Increase Mather. The Byles daughters in Halifax and Saint John grew up in a household known for its intellectual, literary, and theological traditions, and their letters illustrate their ongoing association with their family members remaining in Boston.

to her aunt in a letter in March 1784, was that "our Boys are all intended for the Army or Navy; or some post under Government where neither knowledge or Honesty are required. Indeed they retard a person's advancement; to Dance, make a genteel Bow, fill up a *printed message card,* and sign a receipt for their pay compleat their education and they step forth *accomplished Gentlemen."* With women, it is a different matter, she adds. Under Deborah Cottnam's guidance, "they have the best Education the place affords and the accomplishment of their *minds* is attended to as well as the adorning of their *persons."* With such an education behind them, Rebecca Byles fully expected "in a few years...to see women fill the most important offices in *Church* and *State"* in Nova Scotia."[11]

While Rebecca Byles's optimism was perhaps premature, the ripple effect created by Deborah Cottnam's students was probably very real if reference to former teachers in women's correspondence is indicative of their usual influence. In the case of Deborah Cottnam, this effect extended into the literary sphere as well as the educational one, and she therefore becomes important in representing a certain continuity in the development of women's literary taste in the Maritimes. References in the Byles letters indicate that women of poetic sensibility like the Byles sisters continued to benefit from her friendship and conversation long after leaving her school, and within Deborah Cottnam's own family there is ample evidence of the effect of one generation on the next in developing an appreciation for reading and writing poetry. Employing the pseudonym "Portia," Deborah Cottnam was herself a poet of considerable control and strength. Her elegies "The Mourning Mother" and "Written extempore, on hearing of the death of the Amiable Mrs. Lowell" develop a tension between reason and feeling, and in both poems the speaker seems to be struggling to find purpose in God's will. While a pious acceptance of Divine purpose ultimately predominates in the elegies, there is behind the epigrammatic lines on Mrs. Lowell's death a suggestion that the speaker's submission to God's plan is not without a recognition of its irony: "Blessed with all that Heaven on Earth could give,/ The Power Supreme bid lovely Lowell live;/ Her worth transcending all beneath the sky —/ To crown her virtues — lo! He bids her die!"[12]

Although little of Deborah Cottnam's work has survived, her memory was kept alive in nineteenth-century Nova Scotia by the occasional reprinting of her poem "On Being Asked What Recollection Was." Illustrating a less formal side of her writing in both its subject matter and its style, the poem is

---

10 R. Byles, "My ever Dear Aunt," 6 January 1779, Byles Collection, MG 1, vol. 163, Folder 3, PANS.

11 R. Byles to her aunt, 24 March 1784, *ibid.*

12 Portia, "Written Extempore, On Hearing of the Death of the Amiable Mrs. Lowell," *The Novascotian,* "Nights with the Muses, No. 4," 16 June 1845.

an address to a young lady whose question becomes the unifying motif of the work. It is a tender poem and, in its thoughtful endeavour to answer Eliza's query to the best of the speaker's ability, reveals Deborah Cottnam in the role of teacher and parent as well as poet. After exploring a series of possible definitions, the poet gracefully brings the poem back to the individual who was the source of the exercise: "To explain what baffles all descriptive arts — / The *Deity* implanted in our hearts;/ Struck and convinced, I drop the onequal [*sic*] task,/ Nor further dare though *my Eliza ask.*"[13]

The continuity in taste and interest that was passed on from one generation of daughters to the next in the Cottnam family is illustrated by the literary interests of Deborah Cottnam's daughter, Martha Cottnam Tonge, and by the emergence of her great-granddaughter in the 1820s as one of Nova Scotia's most promising young poets. Of Martha Cottnam Tonge's literary output almost nothing remains, but a recorded fragment of her verse suggests that she was a private poet,[14] who resembled her friend, Rebecca Byles, in preferring to circulate her work among her friends rather than publish it abroad.[15]

---

13 Portia, "On Being Asked What Recollection was," *ibid.*; reprinted in *The Provincial, Or Halifax Monthly Magazine*, "Half Hour with Our Poets," January 1852, pp. 46-47 [without its final lines]; reprinted (abridged) in *The Acadian Recorder*, "Occasional's Letter," 15 March 1919.

14 In *The Novascotian*, "Nights with the Muses," 23 June 1845, there is a fragment of Martha Cottnam Tonge's verse. Written in an album and published posthumously, the lines are introduced by a brief salutation:

Mrs. Tonge and her fire-side circle return this book with thanks for the indulgence of a perusal:

> While in these pages, pleased, we find
> True taste and judgement well, combined
> With native elegance of mind —
>   From us what should you fear?
> We, quite unskilled in rules of art,
> With carping critics take no part —
> But verse which gently melts the heart,
>   To us is ever dear.

These lines seem to emphasize the private nature of Mrs. Tonge's work.

15 R. Byles to Miss Kitty Byles, 1 June 1785, Byles Collection, MG 1, Vol. 163, Folder 3, PANS. In this letter, Rebecca suggests that the modesty of women writers may make them shy away from exposing their work to "the free censures, the ill natur'd criticisms of one sex, the envy and jealousy of the other." She acknowledges, "myself by no means an advocate for a woman's ever exposing her Writings to the publick Eye." While not wanting to limit women, she can but think that "a woman would never wish them [her writings], to go beyond the circle of her intimate connexions." The prevalence of this attitude no doubt explains the dearth of women's writing appearing in the newspapers in the late eighteenth century.

However, through her influence, the literary interests of Deborah Cottnam were kept alive in the next two generations of the family, a fact acknowledged by her great-granddaughter, Griselda Tonge, in her commemorative poem, "To My Dear Grandmother, On her 80th Birth Day." Published on 5 March 1825 in *The Acadian Recorder* (Halifax), the poem is ostensibly a tribute to Martha Cottnam Tonge, but significantly it begins with a recognition of Deborah Cottnam's literary influence on the speaker. In doing so, it suggests a creative tradition that has been passed down through successive generations of women in the family:

> How oft from honoured Certia's [sic; Portia's] polished lyre
> In tones harmonious this loved theme has flowed;
> Each strain, while breathing all the poet's fire
> The feeling heart and fertile fancy showed;
> Oftimes in childhood my young mind has glowed
> While dwelling on her sweet descriptive lay —
> Oh, that on me the power had been bestowed!
> A tribute fitting for the theme to pay,
> With joy I'd touch each string to welcome in this day.[16]

While Griselda Tonge modestly laments in this poem that "power" has not been "bestowed" from great-grandmother to great-granddaughter, the evidence points to the cultivation of literary interests and a sense of literary unity in the family for over 50 years. It would be gratifying to find examples of such unity among a broader spectrum of writing women in Nova Scotia before 1850, but a paucity of records makes such a generalization impossible. Nonetheless, in the family literary tradition sustained by the daughter and great-granddaughter of Deborah Cottnam and in the standards of taste passed down through the graduates of schools like hers, there are indications of how a subculture of women's literature and influence could develop and be sustained within the cultural mainstream of early Nova Scotia.

The literary success of Deborah Cottnam's great-granddaughter was unfortunately short-lived, for in 1825 Griselda Tonge died of fever while visiting her brother in Demerara in the West Indies. She had been one of the most promising of the women writers who in the 1820s began to augment the private circulation of their writing with publication in the periodicals and newspapers of the region. Her 1825 poem to her grandmother, published in *The Acadian Recorder* (Halifax), had received the praise of Scottish-born litterateur, James Irving. Irving had commended her handling of the difficult

---

16   "To My Dear Grandmother On Her 80th Birth Day," *The Acadian Recorder*, 5 March 1825. The newspaper erroneously printed "Certia" for "Portia" in line 1 of the first printing of this poem. This was corrected in subsequent reprintings of the poem.

Spenserian stanza form and had paid tribute to her ability to develop a sense of sincere affection in a genre more often characterized by "the cold strains of flattery."[17] Such praise did much to solidify Griselda Tonge's reputation, and on the basis of a small body of work written by the time of her death at twenty, Joseph Howe, Mary Jane Katzmann, William Arthur Calnek, and other Nova Scotian writers continued to extol and even mythologize Griselda Tonge throughout the nineteenth century.[18]

While Griselda Tonge's work won popularity in the 1820s for its poetic control and sincerity, it represented a romanticism in subject matter more frequently found in the poetry of the period than in the prose. Satire and irony preoccupied many of the sketch writers of the decade, with some of the best satire of the early 1820s focusing on the follies and foibles of Halifax society. Among the writers to emerge in the periodical press in these years was the anonymous creator of the "Patty Pry Letters," a series of ironic sketches subtly revealing the indignity suffered by women in a society where marriage is the only option.[19] Set in Halifax in 1826, these ostensible letters to a newspaper editor employ dramatic confrontation, tales within tales, and old correspondence as devices to fill in past history and to put Patty's contemporary story in the context of the previous generation in Ireland. Thus, the author establishes a sense of continuity about women's situation in society, for although Patty in Halifax in the 1820s seems better educated and freer from convention than her Aunt Tabby in Cork 40 years before, she is in fact as bound by the expectations of society as was her relative. In the old country, class considerations thwarted Tabby's chances of happiness and reduced her to relying forever on the benevolent paternalism of her brother. In the new country, Patty has learned to exploit that kind of paternalism and to use her own sexuality to her advantage (she sits on her father's knee, lets him rumple her curls, and allows him to rest his gouty leg on her lap in order to woo him into a relenting humour). However, what is clear to the reader throughout the first-person narration of the sketches is that Patty is in fact two

17 Introduction to *ibid., The Acadian Recorder*, 5 March 1825. James Irving, who wrote the complimentary introduction to Griselda Tonge's poem, was a Scot who immigrated to Nova Scotia around 1819. He wrote for a number of periodicals in Scotland and England, including *The Dumfries and Galloway Courier* and *The Edinburgh Monthly Magazine*. In the 1820s, he wrote criticism, poetry, and essays for *The Acadian Recorder* and *The Acadian Magazine*.

18 See Joseph Howe, *Western and Eastern Rambles: Travel Sketches of Nova Scotia*, ed. M.G. Parks (Toronto, 1973), pp. 66-69; *The Provincial, or Halifax Monthly Magazine*, "Half Hour with Our Poets" (January 1852), pp. 45-49; and W. Arthur Calnek, "Distinguished Canadians," *Stewart's Quarterly*, 4 (October 1870), p. 294.

19 Under the caption "For *The Novascotian*," the letters of Patty Pry appeared in *The Novascotian* from 29 June 1826 until 7 September 1826. They have been reprinted in David Arnason, ed., *Nineteenth Century Canadian Stories* (Toronto, 1976), pp. 33-51.

persons — the mindless pretty coquette who twitters to the editor and her father about her busy day of "dress, dancing, and parties"[20] — and the intelligent young woman who reads LeSage, Shakespeare, Dr. Johnson, and Addison and Steele in her quiet moments. Her observation that love "is the article in which we deal and by which we hope to make our bread"[21] smacks of a certain ironic assessment of her situation, as does her rather cynical remark that on Saturdays "nineteen-twentieths of the ladies are in every Christian country, preparing for the decorations of the Sunday."[22] There is a sense throughout the letters that the narrator has no illusions about her own situation, but feels she must write in the clever slang and breezy tone expected of her public image: "'Tis of no use denying it — I know I did curl up my nose, and looked with queer astonishment at her puckered lips, and at the lank locks which were swagging on her shrivelled cheek. The side of Aunt's cheek is just like the coating of a shrivelled winter apple in June. A pretty puss, thought I, to cry at a love story."[23] By the end of the sketches, however, Patty has learned to sympathize with her aunt and has recognized in her life story the poignancy of individual women in her society.

The author of the "Patty Pry Letters" remains anonymous, but an editor's note in *The Novascotian* (Halifax) on 3 August 1826 suggests that the writer is a woman. It also indicates that the editor deleted material from one of the episodes, but whether this was done to alter style or opinion is unclear. What is clear on surveying the periodical press, however, is that the hypocrisy and paternalism revealed by the "Patty Pry Letters" is rarely exposed in Nova Scotian writing in the 1830 to 1850 period. Instead, characteristic works like Joseph Howe's "The Moral Influence of Women"[24] or Miss Grove's *Little Grace*[25] portray women as happy wives and mothers leading satisfying lives under the beneficent eye of their model, Queen Victoria. Few and far between are the voices of dissent like that of Jane MacPhail of Pictou, an abolitionist whose single copy of *Uncle Tom's Cabin* circulated throughout the community in 1852. Jane MacPhail's letters to her abolitionist friend, Ann

---

20 Patty Pry, "Letter II," *The Novascotian*, 6 July 1826; reprinted in *Nineteenth Century Canadian Stories*, p. 36.

21 Patty Pry, "Letter I," *The Novascotian*, 29 June 1826; reprinted in *Nineteenth Century Canadian Stories*, pp. 33-34.

22 *Ibid.*

23 *Ibid.*; an anonymous light response appears in *The Acadian Recorder*, 22 July 1826.

24 Joseph Howe, "The Moral Influence of Women," Halifax Mechanics' Institute, September 1836; printed in Joseph Howe, *Poems and Essays* (1847; rpt. Toronto, 1973), pp. 248-75.

25 Miss Grove, *Little Grace; or, Scenes in Nova Scotia* (Halifax, 1846). Designed to teach girls the history of Nova Scotia, this book also reinforced Victorian middle-class values and Victorian concepts of womanhood.

Warren Weston[26] of Boston, reveal her frustration in trying to organize Pictou women to assist her in her work against slavery and capital punishment and illustrate her conviction that social and political organizations are a means of liberating women from intellectual and social restrictions:

> Has not the abolition agitation done much for the women of the United States: What would you all have been but for it, amusing yourselves with such toys as men would please to set before you, on "feasting the Parson with the spare-rib" while father, brother, or husband would be toiling at the desk. I never read a soul stirring article from the pen of one of your women, but...the same instrumentality will yet rouse the women of Great Britain into a proper sense of their position, when they will lay aside childish toys and assume the bearing and attitude of rational beings and of free yet responsible agents and fulfill their high destiny.[27]

Jane MacPhail represented a small socially and politically active group of women in Nova Scotia in the mid-Victorian period, but there is little evidence in the poetry, fiction, and drama published in mid-century that any of these women were interested in giving imaginative expression to their philosophical or social convictions. While Jane MacPhail urged her sex to "lay aside childish toys," the majority of women publishing in Nova Scotia in this period were in fact writing the escapist romances and sentimental poetry which someone of her sensibility deplored. Moreover, by mid-century the opportunities for the publication of such writing had vastly improved for literary women in the province. By 1851, Mary Eliza Herbert had founded *The Mayflower,* a women's periodical that invited regional literary submissions and offered its readers escape into "the flowery fields of romance."[28] Directed at the rising middle-class woman who wanted to know how to organize her servants, how to decorate her home, and how to converse on the latest popular authors, *The Mayflower* seemed to Mary Eliza Herbert to offer a viable alternative to the influx of American women's magazines being circulated in the region. Too modest to compete with the tinted plates and fashion fold-outs in *Godey's Ladies Book, The Mayflower* nonetheless offered the Maritime woman an opportunity to read regional material as well

---

26 Ann Warren Weston (1812-90) was a leader in the Boston Female Anti-Slavery Society. She and her sister, Deborah, helped organize the bazaars which raised money for the cause. Jane McPhail of Pictou sent Micmac craft work to the bazaars in the 1840s and the early 1850s in an effort to assist the work of the Boston women.

27 Jane McPhail to Miss Weston, 29 June 1852, Canadian Collection, Rare Books, Boston Public Library.

28 Editorial, *The Mayflower,* I (May 1851), p. 29.

as that from Great Britain and the United States, and it gave women the possibility of being published when they wrote on subjects compatible with the spirit of the magazine.

Rather surprisingly, the Methodist church supported Mary Eliza Herbert's venture into "the flowery fields of romance," commending the fact that *The Mayflower* would give Maritime women an outlet for their writing while affording them an opportunity to learn new information. Whether the church supported the young editor because of her own impeccable Methodist background,[29] or whether it saw the journal as endorsing the family values, temperance views, and feminine self-education that were part of the Methodist canon, is difficult to say, but the official organ of the church, *The Wesleyan Magazine,* did not moralize as might be expected about the frivolity of *The Mayflower's* publishing sentimental fiction. However, Mary Eliza Herbert obviously did encounter criticism of this nature from some religious sources, for in her editorial of August 1851 she discussed the problem of "good-meaning people" who put "all works of imagination, except those of decidedly religious character, in an unfavourable light."[30] While not alluding to the situation as a personal one, she went on to argue "that well written works of imagination, of a moral and intellectual character, may not only be harmless but positively beneficial" in their ability to stimulate those disinclined to read a religious or moral essay.[31]

Although Mary Eliza Herbert may have expected (and did receive) criticism from conservative religious groups who sanctioned periodicals only if they elevated the spirit, she did not expect controversy over the execution and integrity of the journal. It was a surprise, therefore, when in May and June of 1851 the Reverend James Cochran, Anglican editor of *The Church Times* (Lunenburg), attacked *The Mayflower* for its poor typography, meagreness of original material, and lack of grace and elegance. Objecting to its overall impression of "cheapness," he imputed motives of profit to the

---

29 Born in Halifax in 1829, Mary Eliza Herbert was baptized in Old Zoar Chapel by the renowned Methodist clergyman, Bishop William Black, and spent a lifetime closely associated with the Methodist Church. She contributed poetry and sketches to *The Wesleyan Magazine* and to the newspapers, and in the years following the demise of *The Mayflower* in 1852 published a volume of poetry, *The Aeolian Harp* (1857), and three novels. Like her half-sister Sarah, Mary Eliza Herbert taught Sabbath School and supported the efforts of the Temperance Society (their father, an Irish-born shoemaker and blacking manufacturer in Halifax, was the Grand Conductor of The Sons of Temperance in the late 1850s). The stress on piety in Mary Eliza Herbert's background seems to have inhibited her imaginative development as a writer, for she invariably sacrificed vivid characterization and humour to the demands of a moral and uplifting conclusion.

30 Mary E. Herbert, "Works of Imagination," *The Mayflower,* I (August 1851), p. 125.

31 *Ibid.,* p. 126.

editor and criticized the quality of the paper as being unsuitable for the "parlour or boudoir."[32]

Germane to an understanding of this attack is the realization that James Cochran was a man of aesthetic tastes. However, plain and unexciting as the graphic layout of Mary Eliza Herbert's periodical was, it was not an incompetently-produced publication. Thus, it is also relevant to the issue to consider the Reverend Cochran's comment that *The Mayflower* was too unattractive in appearance to grace the "parlour or boudoir." Clearly, one of the issues at stake in *The Church Times* attack on *The Mayflower* was the different image of women that each magazine and its editor endorsed. An Anglican gentleman of the old school, Cochran was to give a public address in Halifax in 1864 in which his concept of womanhood was clearly articulated:

> Yes, old man and minister as I am, I hope I may be allowed to say that every time I meet these daughters of Acadia I feel proud of them — I love to see their bright eyes, their rosy cheeks, their cheerful smiles — Whatever they are — R.C., Ch. Dissenters, high or low I love them all — They make us good wives, good mothers, good daughters, good sisters — as any country under the sun can boast of. Nor is literary talent wanting among them. They can write poetry as sweet to mouth, and stories as pathetic as need be read.[33]

To Cochran, women were sensitive, cheerful creatures who gladdened the male heart in their domestic and artistic devotion. It is perhaps not surprising, therefore, that a plain little magazine run by the efficient daughter of an Irish Methodist shoemaker should seem slightly plebeian to the reverend gentleman. To emphasize just where plebeianism in fact lay, Mary Eliza Herbert launched a spirited counter-attack on Cochran in July 1851. Responding to his charge that *The Mayflower* lacked a large body of original material, she argued that many of the most pretentious and opinionated journals of the day had a poor record of publishing local literature. Lest *The Church Times* escape the meaning of her allusion, she went on to openly attack Cochran for his suggestion that remuneration might be her chief consideration:

> He "trusts, however, that the Mayflower will be remunerative, which is, he dares say, the *chief consideration.*" Of course he is free from all desire of being remunerated for his own efforts to cater for the public. We dare say he is quite disinterested, otherwise he would not know so

---

32 James Cochran, "Untitled Editorial," *The Church Times*, 20 June 1851.
33 James Cochran, "Recollections of Half a Century" (1864), p. 32n, Vertical Mss. File, PANS.

well to impute motives to others. His reference to the "chief consideration," we regard as altogether beneath serious notice. When he informs us of his *gratuitous* labors for the public enlightenment, we shall give him due credit for being a genuine philanthropist; but until that auspicious moment shall have arrived, he will not take it amiss if we remind him that silence on "the chief consideration" will better become him than ungentlemanly allusions.[34]

Mary Eliza Herbert shrewdly turned the tables on Cochran when she accused him of ungentlemanly behaviour, and after her sally, the attacks from *The Church Times* stopped. However, *The Mayflower's* troubles did not cease at this point, and it was clear by the summer of 1851 that, without a larger subscription list, its founder could not sustain the journal at its inexpensive price of 7s.6d per annum. Moreover, the creative contributions she had expected from the women writers of the province never materialized in the quantity desired. Trying to provide a balanced blend of American, British, and regional works, she had to rely more and more on her own resources. Poems, essays, and novellas *(Emily Linwood, or, The Bow of Promise* and *Ambrose Mandeville)* appeared in the journal under her recognized soubriquet "M.E.H.," "M.," and "H.," but the copy of *The Mayflower* in the Baldwin Room of the Toronto Public Library suggests that she wrote far more for *The Mayflower* than previously has been realized. The pseudonyms "T.R.," "Anon.," "Marion," "E.," "W.R.," and "Len" have all been crossed out in the Baldwin Room copy and "M.E.H." has been written in the margin in what seems to be Mary Eliza Herbert's hand. Thus, it seems possible from this particular volume of the journal that financial exigencies and a dearth of regional contributions forced Mary Eliza Herbert into the position of writing nearly all the indigenous content of *The Mayflower* herself while pretending to the public that she held a balance between selected and regional material. In so doing, she changed the character of the magazine from being an illustration of women's literary activity in the Maritimes in the early 1850s to being instead a reflection of her own creative skills.

The Mayflower collapsed in February 1852. It had not been a reforming journal, but it had assumed that women were both intelligent and efficient. This impression had been supported by Mary Eliza Herbert's own fiction published in the magazine, for in spite of giving pious, "happy-ever-after" endings to her stories, she had always portrayed her heroines as being self-reliant, hard-working, and indifferent to class distinctions. An educated heart invariably brought the Herbert protagonists their just reward, although in the years following the demise of *The Mayflower,* the author occasionally created a fictional world where destiny played cruel tricks on her heroines. One such

---

34   Mary E. Herbert, "Notices of *The Mayflower," The Mayflower,* I (July 1851), p. 93.

story is *Belinda Dalton, or Scenes in The Life of a Halifax Belle* (1859), a novel of manners and morals set in contemporary Halifax. Mary Eliza Herbert reveals a flair for dramatic dialogue and an ability to create strong minor characters in this work, but her talents are undercut by the necessity of focusing the novel on the pious (and, therefore, dull) Belinda. Nonetheless, Belinda is not a totally conventional heroine in the author's canon. When Belinda's fiancé dies, she prefers a life of spinsterhood to a marriage of convenience. Alone in old age, she finds herself outside the mainstream of society. While her memories and her virtuous heart sustain her somewhat, she illustrates the predicament of women who are educated for domestic life but not for the realities of managing their own financial affairs. Lawyer Levit unscrupulously swindles Belinda out of all her property in exchange for "a hundred pounds to meet your present difficulties, and a life annuity of twenty-five pounds, with the use of two apartments in one of the dwellings."[35] Proud but impoverished at the end of the novel, Belinda walks the streets in her rusty black garb and alleviates loneliness by doing good deeds. Her story, notes the author in her moralistic last paragraph, is a lesson to all those who will "speak in a somewhat contemptuous tone, of that often unjustly despised class, old maids...." In Belinda's tale lies an illustration of the fact "that virtue is not incompatible with poverty, and that the friendless are those who should most fully share in the sympathies of the youthful heart."[36]

Mary Eliza Herbert was not interested in writing a novel with social overtones when she published *Belinda Dalton, or Scenes in The Life of a Halifax Belle,* and the work therefore lacks the impact which a more sociologically inclined writer might have given it. That Herbert may have had the ability to write such a work, however, is suggested by her manuscript novel, *Lucy Cameron,* now lodged in the Dalhousie University Archives. Like Belinda Dalton, Lucy Cameron presents the situation of a woman who does not want to marry merely for the purpose of gaining security. However, Lucy does not inherit money as does Belinda, and she lacks the requisite education for securing a teaching position. Genteel in her tastes but penniless and without family, she is forced into a marriage of convenience for economic reasons. The narrator's portrait of this marriage and of Lucy's businessman husband is unsubtle but relentless in its exposure of marriage as a form of middle-class investment:

> As Lucy took her seat at the head of the table and presided with gentle grace, at the bountiful and well-served repast, Mr. Cameron's dull grey

---

35 Mary E. Herbert, *Belinda Dalton; or, Scenes in the Life of a Halifax Belle* (Halifax, 1859), p. 58.

36 *Ibid.,* p. 60.

eyes rested upon her with a gleam of satisfaction, and a thrill of pride and pleasure swelled his heart, that he had secured, as the mistress of his home, one so well fitted to adorn it. A shrewd businessman, he had, nevertheless, indulged what fancy he possesed [sic] in the selection of a wife, and he loved her as much as his cold, worldly, ambitious nature had room to spare.

He compared her with the wives of his acquaintances and friends, and assuredly she lost nothing by the comparison. What were they? pretty dolls, not much more, only good for fashion, and flirtation and nonsense, drawling out a meagre "yes" or "no," if you tried them on any sensible subject; now, *his* could converse, and well, too; really he was proud of her, but prouder of himself for obtaining her.

You perceive that this man thought only of himself; he saw he had made a good bargain, and rejoiced in it, but in all his musings, he never troubled himself about his wife's view of the matter, or if, for a moment, he dwelt on it, it was to suppose how deeply grateful she must be for the affluent circumstances in which he had placed her, as contrasted with her earlier surroundings.[37]

Balancing the reader's insight into the husband's reflections are the moments when the narrator reveals Lucy's hours of relentless soul-searching. Examining the state of her bargain and her marriage, she is aware that she represents nothing more than another contract. The most galling thing for her is that she has signed this financial arrangement with the devil herself:

"If he were only my brother, cousin, Uncle, anything else but my husband," she broke out passionately; "but to know that I belong to him, that I have forged, with my own hands, life-long fetters, to read in every look, in every action, that he considers me his property; one whose sole aim should be to cheer, amuse, and minister to him, a 'Something dearer than his dog and nobler than his horse,' ah this is bitterness indeed."[38]

What *Lucy Cameron* reminds one of are the feminist sensation-novels of the 1860s and 1870s in Britain, particularly Rhoda Broughton's *Cometh Up As a Flower* (1867), where another motherless girl marries for security and is subsequently wracked by self-contempt as she views the hopelessness of her

---

37 Mary Eliza Herbert, *Lucy Cameron*, Ms. 2.32, Folders 8-10, (Halifax n.d.), Dalhousie University Archives.

38 *Ibid.*, Folders 13-14.

contract. Nell in Broughton's novel is finally released from her bondage by dying of consumption. Herbert's Lucy Cameron suffers a more palatable fate. Mr. Cameron eventually dies and the novel concludes with Lucy (now financially secure) meeting her childhood sweetheart and marrying him.

Although Mary Eliza Herbert gave *Lucy Cameron* a sentimental ending as an antidote to its frank passages, she never published the novel. It is interesting to speculate why she did not, for her drive to authorship resulted in her publishing nearly everything she wrote. It is possible that she thought Lucy Cameron's confessions might provoke the kind of protest that Rhoda Broughton's novel created in England. She may also have been concerned about shocking her usual readership, an audience which hitherto had been reassured of the rightness of its world when it read a Herbert story. The other possibility is that the novel was not finished to the author's satisfaction before tuberculosis cut her life short in 1872. No papers, letters, or financial records survive from Mary Eliza Herbert's ventures, so much about her professional life and attitudes lies in the realm of conjecture. In *Lucy Cameron,* however, there is at least a suggestion that Mary Eliza Herbert had inclinations in writing women's fiction which she found it expedient to suppress in the small and conservative literary market of the Maritimes.

In looking at Herbert's writing environment, there is no sense of any solidarity among the women publishing at the time except, perhaps, among the women of Methodist persuasion. The commonplace book of A.M. Valentine now on microfilm in the Public Archives of Nova Scotia suggests that in their youth Maria Morris, Sarah Herbert, Mary Eliza Herbert, and A.M. Valentine all wrote poetry and probably discussed and shared their work.[39] Almira Bell, a dissenting schoolteacher from Barrington, was peripheral to this group because of geography, but she did contribute to their literary activities by sending poetry to *The Mayflower*. Their bond was as much a religious one as a creative one, however, and it is probable that their literary association did not survive the incursions which death and personal circumstances made upon it in the 1840s and 1850s. Otherwise, Mary Eliza Herbert seems to have had few contacts with other literary women of the region, especially those like May Agnes Fleming of Saint John and Mary Jane Katzmann of Halifax, who shared her aspirations for a public writing career. Katzmann resembled Herbert in wanting to create a literary periodical as an outlet for the local writing community, but it is perhaps symptomatic of the lack of coordination between the women writers of the early 1850s that she and Mary Eliza Herbert tried to publish their journals in the limited market of Halifax at approximately the same time.

One reason for Mary Jane Katzmann's reluctance to share periodical publishing with Mary Eliza Herbert might have been the very different

---

39   A.M. Valentine, "Verses," microfilm, MG 1-Biography, PANS.

concept of a literary journal which each endorsed. Herbert wanted to publish especially for women and favoured "the flowery fields of romance." Katzmann, on the other hand, wanted a journal that would inform and stimulate the reader. Her *The Provincial, or Halifax Monthly Magazine* first appeared in January 1852 as a 40-page monthly concentrating on travel descriptions, regional vignettes, informal essays, dialogues, plays, and fictionalized sketches. In one sense, Mary Jane Katzmann was a latter day Sam Slick, for she used her journal to rouse Maritimers to the economic and industrial possibilities of their region. She was also deeply interested in awakening a sense of local history in her audience, and her publication of Native legends, Maritime authors, and local colour tales in *The Provincial, or Halifax Monthly Magazine* did much to confirm for Maritimers that they had culturally come of age. However, like Mary Eliza Herbert, Mary Jane Katzmann ran into financial difficulties with her periodical. She had promised contributing authors remuneration once circulation reached a thousand, but in her last editorial in December 1853, she indicated she was still 100 subscribers short of economic viability. A letter from her printer, J. Bowes and Son, to Elkanah Morton of Halifax in October 1853, gives costs for 500 copies of the journal,[40] and it is very possible Katzmann was anticipating retrenchment at this time. What she clearly was not anticipating in her December 1853 editorial was the cessation of the magazine. However, the December issue was her last, and what seems clear now from the Morton-Bowes correspondence is that Morton, Mary Jane Katzmann's brother-in-law, was the main financial backer of her venture. At this time, Elkanah Morton was constructing an expensive, brick office building in Halifax, and, pressed for funds himself, he in all likelihood withdrew his financial support from his sister-in-law's journal. She subsequently opened a bookstore in Halifax and continued to contribute poetry to periodicals after her marriage in 1868. However, she never again ventured into as ambitious a project as *The Provincial, or Halifax Monthly Magazine* had been, although the awarding of King's College's Akins Historical Prize to her in 1887 gave evidence of the esteem in which her historical work and her writing were held. Mary Jane Katzmann was an Anglican from a genteel family in Halifax and moved in Church of England literary circles. History and literature occupied her attention and at no time did she ever exhibit a concern with the condition or future of her sex in society. Mary Eliza Herbert's interests, on the other hand, were Methodist, domestic, and romantic. To all appearances, it seems that social and religious differences in their two backgrounds gave them little in common. However, they shared mutual frustrations in trying to conduct professional writing and publishing careers in Nova Scotia in the pre-

---

40   J. Bowes & Son to G.E. Morton, Esq., 10 October 1853, Forrest Collection, MG 1, vol. 315, Folder 4. PANS.

Confederation period. Without a dependable financial base, women could not survive as writers in such a small marketplace as the Maritimes proved to be before 1867. Perhaps shrewder or more practical than her contemporaries and predecessors, May Agnes Fleming of Saint John sent her fiction to New York and Boston periodicals in the 1860s. When she married in the 1870s, she left the region for New York. There she cemented relationships with publishers which had begun years before with her magazine publishing. Writing for the market, as Mary Eliza Herbert and Mary Jane Katzmann never did, and demanding fifteen percent royalties from major houses, she was making $10,000 per annum at the same time that Mary Eliza Herbert was publishing her novels at her own expense and trying to sell them at a small profit.[41]

As always, conquering the economics of writing and publishing proved to be more than half the battle, and in the very business-like arrangements that May Agnes Fleming made with publishers in the United States and that Susanna Moodie made with Bentley's in London, there was some guarantee of visibility and distribution if not always of posterity.[42] With the women writers who stayed at home in a pocket culture such as the Maritime area was before 1867, there was no distribution and no lasting fame. Newspapers and periodicals were thrown out when they were read. Letters and financial records were destroyed when the writers died. The result is that we do not know what Deborah Cottnam, Griselda Tonge, Mary Eliza Herbert, or Mary Jane Katzmann thought of themselves as writers, what their ambitions were, how they supported themselves financially, or who bought their writing. Furthermore, because of the circumstances of their publishing, they have been dismissed and forgotten in the writing of our literary histories — modest foothills, as Eggleston's thesis goes, lying in the shadow of mountains.

---

41 "Mrs. May Agnes Fleming," *News* (Saint John), 14 December 1878; clipping held in Anonymous Scrapbooks, 0-Vol. 1, p. 215, Saint John Free Library.

42 At the beginning of Susanna Moodie's publishing career with Richard Bentley & Son of London, she negotiated favourable terms through her agent, John Bruce of Dorset (for example, rights to reprint her work in Canada after ten years or an advance of from 20 to 50 pounds on profits which would not have to be repaid if the book did not sell). Her arrangements with Bentley did not prevent her from negotiating separately with American publishers. With the success of *Roughing it in The Bush, or, Forest Life in Canada,* in 1852, Bentley sent Susanna Moodie 50 pounds more "as a compliment beyond the consideration for the copyright of *Roughing It in The Bush.*" (Richard Bentley to Mrs. Moodie, 11 August 1852, The Archives of Richard Bentley & Son: 1829-1898, Reel 40, vol. 82, p. 237, British Library, London). As the taste for Susanna Moodie's kind of writing declined, however, the arrangements with Bentley became less generous (although no less cordial). That Susanna Moodie carefully watched her financial arrangements with her publisher is clear in a letter of 10 February 1854, when Bentley notes "how particular you are in your arrangements with me as to pecuniary matters" (Richard Bentley to Mrs. Moodie, 10 February 1854, *ibid.,* p. 371).

The Club Papers:
Haliburton's Literary Apprenticeship

As D.C. Harvey has pointed out in "The Intellectual Awakening of Nova Scotia," the period after 1812 saw the establishment of academies, newspapers, libraries, reading societies, and other institutions that encouraged the development of an indigenous culture in the province.[1] The publication of Agricola's essays in 1818-21,[2] Thomas McCulloch's "Stepsure" letters in 1821-23,[3] James Irving's "Letters on The Present State of English Poetry" in 1820-22,[4] and a body of satirical newspaper sketches between 1818 and 1825, all complemented activity in other fields and gave evidence of an emerging literary sensibility in the province. "We of this province cannot boast of many golden dreams and speculations, but we are advancing in the course of improvement at a steady, solid pace," wrote Judge J.A. Stewart to his friend Peleg Wiswall in 1825; "Everything shows this — Our trade, our agriculture, our revenue, our population, our tranquillity and contentment, speak a strong language, not in favour of rapid wealth and prosperity, but of gradual and permanent benefit."[5] It was this climate of tempered optimism and economic growth that quickened the intellect and confidence of young Nova Scotians, noted Harvey, and provided the appropriate financial and social base whereby literary endeavour and cultural expression could be nourished.[6]

Characteristic of the literary activity of this period was the emergence of a series of satirical sketches first published in Joseph Howe's *The Novascotian* on 8 May 1828, and continued in the journal at intermittent intervals until 12

---

1 D.C. Harvey, "The Intellectual Awakening of Nova Scotia" in G.A. Rawlyk, ed., *Historical Essays on the Atlantic Provinces* (Toronto, 1967).

2 John Young's ("Agricola") essays on agriculture appeared in *The Acadian Recorder* from 1818-21 and were published in book form under the title *The Letters of Agricola on the Principles of Vegetation and Tillage* (Halifax, 1822). Agricola continued to contribute articles on agriculture to the newspapers in 1823.

3 Thomas McCulloch's anonymous Stepsure letters appeared in *The Acadian Recorder* from 22 December 1821 to 29 March 1823. In their satire on Nova Scotians' failure to work hard and develop the land, they anticipated Thomas Chandler Haliburton's better-known Sam Slick sketches.

4. James Irving's "Letters on the Present State of English Poetry" began to appear in *The Acadian Recorder* on 13 May 1820 and continued to be published at regular intervals for the next two years. They set a standard for literary criticism in the province and generated much discussion on literary matters.

5 J.A. Stewart to Peleg Wiswall, 21 March 1825, Wiswall Collection, MG 1, Vol. 980, Folder 11, Number 100, Public Archives of Nova Scotia (PANS).

6 Harvey, "Intellectual Awakening," p. 116.

October 1831. Ostensibly celebrating the meetings of a society of gentlemen gathered in a Halifax chamber for good conversation, good port, and the taste of a fine Havana, the 52 satires, songs, dialogues, and dramas appeared under the simple designation, "The Club". Always consisting of at least four people, this pseudonymous body would meet secretly in a snug room well removed from the public eye. Here, protected and pampered by a doorman named Ponsonby, the members would argue far into the night on subjects as varied as literary theory, political preferment, provincial history, country living, female education, and the Peninsular Wars. With its fellowship composed of such fictitious Halifax stalwarts as Major Metheglin of the British army; Frank Haliday, an idealistic young lawyer; Ned Barrington, a lovesick poet; and Dr. Febres, a caustic medical man, the Club would occasionally add to its numbers such new recruits as Mr. Editor (Joseph Howe of *The Novascotian),* Mr. Merlin, and Morgan Rattler. From time to time it would also entertain such casual visitors as Peter Pink, Mr. Homer, Donald MacGregor, and Mr. Marlow. The result was a boisterous, roistering company of the bowl, a gathering of gentlemen supposedly bound by no rules except those of courtesy and good fellowship with "no object save amusement."[7]

In spite of the Club's stated dedication to folly and fun, it was obvious from the very beginning of the series that the Club's humour was to be as socially relevant as it was enjoyable. Exposing "vice and folly" and "the heedless race,"[8] the Club was to make class inequality, colonial patronage, upward mobility, religious persecution, and educational discrimination all targets of sharp observation. When John Alexander Barry, the Member for Shelburne County, was dismissed from the House in 1829 and was imprisoned for contempt, the Club was to conduct a mock inquisition, interrogating everyone from Thomas Chandler Haliburton to the Speaker of the House to determine areas of responsibility in the scandal. When Edmund Ward of *The Free Press* took one of his well-known positions of intransigency in his newspaper, the Major was to charge dramatically into the Club-room on a braying ass named Neddy. And when Dr. Thomas McCulloch and the funding of his Pictou Academy dominated the legislature, the Club authors were to reduce the controversy between Secessionists, Kirkmen, and the Council to the level of farce, creating in Donald MacGregor's vision of an assault on Pictou Academy an image so exaggerated that it reduced the paranoia and emotionalism surrounding the issue to the level of the ridiculous:

> . . . the Academy will first be stormed and demolished and the bottles o'lightnin' and the jars o'fermentation, and a' the apparatus for the

---

7   "The Club," *The Novascotian* (Halifax), 8 May 1828.

8   *Ibid.,* 15 June 1831.

black art, broken, and in the vera place whar the Doctor's butterflys are noo pinn'd against the wa', his sons and doghters will be stickit wi' bayonets and ither things; and the puir little body, Cunnabel, gin he na' rin up Jacob's ladder, or some ither braw contrivance, will be crammed into the mou' o' a muckle gun, and blawn whar his wits winna be early come at. When the fecht is gained, as ye may well suppose, there will be nae lack o' bonfires and burnings, violations of person and property — many a bonny lass wha wad hae looked blate at the sight o' a man, will be obligated to sit on his knee; and mony an auld women — (*Haliday*, interrupting him, " Oh! surely the old ladies will be spared.") Wisht mon, wisht, ye'll pit me out. And mony an auld woman whose stock o' cheese an sneeshin' wad hae lasted a year and a day, will na' hae a rind or a dust to comfort her nose or her stomach.[9]

In short, the role of the Club was to provoke and protect —to expose hypocrisy and irrationality in Nova Scotian society and "without fear, favor or affectation...watch over the interest of the world."[10] Intimate with provincial society and politics because of their professional status, and at the same time distanced from it by their ironic vision and anonymity, the Club members seemed well cast to don the cloak of moral indignation and authority so characteristic of many of the sketches. The group was, in fact, the self-proclaimed conscience of Nova Scotia, seeing "the whole population of the province...turning their eyes toward the Club for counsel and protection."[11] Should the fellowship ever disband, noted the Major, Halifax would "run riot for want of proper censorship."[12] For that reason it was often his dramatic function in the series to reiterate the aims and responsibilities of the Club, thereby not only lending literary unity to the sketches by acting as spokesman for the group but also restating for the general reader of *The Novascotian* the importance of the series in exposing both the public and private idiocies of their time:

Did not my heart gladden, although far away [London], to hear the responsive echoes which the province sent back, from time to time, to the patriotic and fearless sentiments you breathed; did I not feel that this Club, like the club of Hercules, although it may sometimes lose an old knot like myself, is still all powerful and matchless upon the earth? This Club, like the King never dies; it may meet in secret or in the open glare of day — its voice may not be heard for months and years —

9   *Ibid.*, 15 May 1828.
10 *Ibid.*, 7 May 1829.
11 *Ibid.*
12 *Ibid.*, 4 February 1830.

mushrooms and toadstools may spring up upon the surface of society; and jackasses may be heard to bray in high and low places, in an idiotic consciousness of its dissolution; but when they least expect its revivification, the former are trampled under its foot, and its lash is applied to the backs of the latter, until they yell like the monster Caliban when the spells of Prospero were upon him.[13]

That jackasses did bray and Calibans did yell under the lash of the Club's wit in *The Novascotian* emerges in the responses of its rival newspapers. "I do not wish to enter into any kind of controversy with you," noted "A Traveller" in an address to Joseph Howe in *The Acadian Recorder*, "particularly as I have a pretty fair specimen of what abuse I may expect from the pen of such an able scurrilist."[14] Nevertheless, he sallied on, castigating the "redoubted assiduity" of the Club's treatment of the Pictou Academy issue, the very creation of the Club, and the nature of its meetings. Even more forceful in his antipathy to the series was "A Countryman," who in March 1829 questioned the morality of Howe and his newspaper in allowing "five or six columns of fictitious dialogue, for the purpose of affording "an opportunity to scoff at everything serious — ...to introduce *Bacchanalian* songs, and disgorge the overflowings of impurity in language and description, at which modesty dare not look, and decency might well shudder — ...and in fine, to form creatures of...imagination, clothe them in the characters of quacks, bullys, pimps, drunkards, and demons, and then make them the Arbiters of public opinion...."[15]

The vehemence of such responses undoubtedly reassured the Club of the full measure of its success and encouraged its continuing existence as the scourge of fools and the bane of "Knaves and imposters who shrink from the shafts of its wit."[16] However, because of the anonymity of the Club body, it was Joseph Howe who invariably bore the brunt of the injured and indignant worthies who responded to the sketches. As editor of *The Novascotian* and as a thinly disguised character in the series, he was perceived by the public to be both the inspiration and the catalyst behind the Club proceedings. That this assumption was not far from the truth is suggested by the correlation between Howe's personal activities and the Club's pattern of appearance in his newspaper. An examination of *The Novascotian* between 1828 and 1831 reveals that when Howe was travelling the province for subscriptions or when he was publishing his "Western" and "Eastern Rambles" in its columns, there

13 *Ibid.*, 1 September 1830.
14 "A Traveller," Letter to Joseph Howe, *The Acadian Recorder*, 7 June 1828.
15 "A Countryman," Letter to Mr. Holland, *ibid.*, 14 March 1829.
16 "Grand Pantomime," *The Novascotian*, 13 January 1830.

was a marked absence of Club material appearing as well.[17] However, when Howe was resident in Halifax and when the city was alive with Assembly meetings and legislative debates, the Club papers appeared at regular intervals, often focusing on political issues in the week's business or responding to current fashions or events. What this seems to suggest is that there were two catalysts in the creation of the sketches — Howe as the organizational force behind the writing and publication of the series, and the sitting of the House as a stimulus for the Club's hypothetical meetings and discussions. As a newspaperman and a budding commentator, Howe undoubtedly recognized the potential the Club afforded him in commenting on current political and social issues, a point reinforced in the sketches themselves when the Major defines it as the duty of the group to meet "at or about the same period of time with the other great Bodies to whom are committed the guidance and government of the world" and to react accordingly in "counteracting the effects of either or all of their measure(s)."[18] However, the sitting of the House also assisted Howe in the development of the Club series in another way, for the meeting of the legislature ensured the presence in Halifax of a large body of eclectic and often talented members from all over the province. Thus, in addition to his regular circle of friends in the city, such as the poet-blacksmith, Andrew Shiels; the British military officer, Captain John Kincaid; the Scottish doctor, William Grigor; and the clever wit and lawyer, Laurence O'Connor Doyle, Howe could add to his coterie during the sitting of the House such literarily-inclined Assemblymen and companions as Thomas Chandler Haliburton (Annapolis) and Jotham Blanchard (Pictou). While not all of these men would be involved in the Club at any given time, they represent the imaginative and literary forces Howe could draw upon at various points over the three years of the series and illustrate the diversity of experience that enabled Howe to sustain the tone and variety of the Club illusion for as long as he did.

The exact process whereby the Club papers were composed and the actual composition of the Howe gatherings at any given time have never been fully discovered. As G.E. Fenety has pointed out in his *Life and Times of the Hon. Joseph Howe*, "the authorship of those 'Club' articles was as profound a secret as that which enshrouded the Junius letters;...and it is doubtful if any

---

17   Howe travelled for the newspaper in the good weather (June-July 1828; June-July and August-October 1829; May-July 1831) and published the "Western Rambles" from 23 July to 9 October 1828. The "Eastern Rambles" appeared from 17 December 1829 to 19 October 1831. The Club Papers usually appeared during the winter-spring term of the House of Assembly. Only in 1830 and on a few occasions in 1831 did any club material appear in the same relative time period as did the "Rambles."

18   "The Club," *The Novascotian*, 1 January 1829.

one outside the printing office ever knew the writer, or writers."[19] Within the sketches themselves, however, there is an image of Mr. Editor and his friends sitting in comfortable surroundings, quaffing their port around the fire, warming their feet upon the fender, and turning the air blue with their good Havanas and their witticisms. The picture is an inviting one and is given some substance by such drinking songs in Howe's canon as his tribute to Thomas Chandler Haliburton, "Here's a health to thee, Tom...."[20] That being said, it is more likely that the Club sketches were composed in the same way as were a number of *Blackwood*'s "Noctes Ambrosianae" — some by a small group of writers who co-operated in shaping a sketch, some by an editor who put down the remembered wit and merriment of the night before, and some by single individuals who had a vision of the characters and their interaction. The survival of copies of *The Novascotian* with the initials "J H." (Joseph Howe), "L.D." (Laurence O'Connor Doyle), "T.C.H." (Thomas Chandler Haliburton), and "Dr. G." (Dr. Grigor) written by hand at the top of certain sketches[21] does suggest individual authorship at least part of the time, and it is entirely feasible to think of a writer's assuming responsibility for certain themes or episodes of personal interest once the conventions and personalities of the characters had been established. Most of the time, however, Howe probably relied (as did Blackwood) on the efforts of two or three people to develop independently or co-operatively the themes and personalities interwoven into an episode.[22] Thus, while the legend of the Club (and of the *Noctes*) grew up around rumours of wild nights of wit and uncontrollable rounds of punning, the reality probably lay somewhere between this attractive picture of conviviality and the usual organization and co-operation demanded in sustaining a newspaper series.

It is not merely on the level of composition that the similarities between Blackwood's "Noctes Ambrosianae" and the Club papers have been noted,[23]

---

19 G.E. Fenety, *Life and Times of Hon. Joseph Howe* (Saint John, 1896), p. 61.

20 Joseph Howe, "A Toast," *Poems and Essays* (Montreal, 1874), p. 169. See also "The Blue Nose," pp. 145-46.

21 The initials "J.H." [Joseph Howe] appear in *The Novascotian* beside "The Club" of 1 January 1829; a stylized "L.D." [Laurence O'Connor Doyle] is beside the sketch of 29 January 1829; "T.H.C." [Thomas Chandler Haliburton] appears beside 5 February 1829; and "Dr. G." [Dr. Grigor] is beside 12 February 1829. Initials that look like "SOC" or "LOC" appear beside "The Club" of 8 January 1829 [possibly Laurence O'Connor Doyle]. Who wrote the initials in these copies of *The Novascotian* (now on the Canadian Library Association Microfilm) is unknown. The names of the Reverend James Cochran, lawyer Harry King, and Catherine Skinner appear on a number of the newspaper copies of the 1828-30 period, but these particular copies are not signed.

22 Alan L. Strout, "Concerning the *Noctes Ambrosianae*," *Modern Language Notes*, LI (December 1936), p. 501.

23 For examples, see J.W. Longley, *Joseph Howe* (Toronto, 1904), p. 9, and James Roy, *Joseph Howe: A Study In Achievement and Frustration* (Toronto, 1935), p. 45.

for there seems to be little doubt that Howe and his colleagues worked with certain proven conventions from the literary sketch tradition and from Blackwood's Edinburgh series in making their comments on Nova Scotian society and politics. The sketch and the Club genres were old and versatile ones when the Halifax wits turned to them, popular in Great Britain for many years and given a special character by the dramatic masks, journalistic immediacy, and satiric thrust of *The Tatler* and *The Spectator* in the early eighteenth century and *The Noctes* conversations published in *Blackwood's* from 1822 to 1835. That the "Noctes'" conversations were as popular with contemporary colonial readers as with British ones is clear from the frequency of their appearance in Maritime newspapers and from the enduring popularity of *Blackwood's Magazine* in regional subscription libraries. Thus there would be few among the Club's readers who would not be familiar with the "Noctes" conventions and would not recognize the parallels in structure and conception between the 52 Club pieces and the 71 sketches of "Noctes" conversations. Just as the "Noctes'" companions gathered in the privacy of Ambrose's tavern in Edinburgh, so the Club members met in secrecy in an unidentified chamber in central Halifax. Instead of the "Noctes" Ambrose, there was the Club's faithful Ponsonby. For Christopher North, the guiding force behind the Scottish series, there was Mr. Editor, Joseph Howe. And just as the Ettrick Shepherd delighted readers everywhere with his Lallans speech and comic philosophy, so Mr. Merlin from the banks of the Yarrow regaled Nova Scotians with his pungent observations on provincial life and literature, all of it delivered in broad Scots dialect. The parallels continue, but in the boisterous merriment, lively conversational exchanges, and broad range of topics which they covered (from the characteristics of German Romantic poetry to raising chickens), the "Noctes'" and the Club not only suggested a common fellowship of the bowl but also a common eclecticism of interests. Thus, it was a master-stroke of Club inventiveness when two-thirds of the way through the series the Major was cast as an emissary from the eminent publisher and bookseller, Blackwood himself. "Who do you think called to see me the other day?" he writes his fellow Club members from London:

> No less a personage than Old Blackwood the bookseller. I thought the fellow was mad, he treated me with so much deference and respect. After some hesitation he disclosed the object of his visit, by saying that Galt, who, you know was lately in Canada, having brought home a file of the Novascotian, he had read with amazement several numbers of the Club; and as Professor Wilson was getting into years, and O'Doherty had impaired his faculties by hard drinking, he would either pay down a large sum per annum for the copyright of our Reports, or, if the whole Club would remove to Edinburgh, he would use his purse and influence to forward our fortunes and make us ample compensation for every

sacrifice. The Doctor he said he could introduce at once to a most respectable and lucrative practice; Haliday, after his admission to the Scotch Bar should have the entire management of all his law business, and Barrington, when not otherwise engaged might write light articles for Maga at a handsome salary — or publish a volume a year of prose or verse on his own account, which, by the aid of extensive Bookselling connections, he could make eminently profitable. Having disposed of you all, he next, after apologizing for making so free, assured me that, as his politics had always been orthodox and as he had always supported the High Tory interest, he could, merely for an able article at a particular juncture, secure me a Regiment, and perhaps, at no distant day get the Major exalted to the rank of Major General! Faith I roared in his face, and assured him that in one month after I communicated his proposal, our friend the Editor would post off to Scotland, and run him through the body.[24]

Scenes like this one in the Club reveal just how versatile Howe and his fellow writers could be with the "Noctes" pattern, for here they not only subvert literary or critical comparisons with the "Noctes" by anticipating and mocking such approaches, but they also transcend the limitations imposed by the "Noctes" conventions by transforming them into the group's own highly original reversal of the colonial mentality. That the Club continued to reshape the familiar into something uniquely its own is further illustrated as the sketches develop an overall character, for although Howe the public editor was still a man of moderation in this period — according to Murray Beck, his biographer, still assuming "the mien of a judge"[25] — he was nonetheless able to expose humbug by hiding behind the mask created by the Club fiction. In this sense, then, the Club began to diverge sharply from the "Noctes" in yet another way, for as the Club sketches became more committed to exposing the follies of Nova Scotian society, they often introduced a more immediate and local element into their conversations than that found in their prototype.

If an imaginative handling of literary convention played some role in assuring the success of the Club papers, a more significant feature in their achievement was the exceedingly talented body of wits and writers that Howe was able to gather around him over the three-year period of the Club's existence. To some extent, the anonymity of the Club's membership has frustrated attempts to identify opinions and contributions, but popular history has consistently associated the names of Andrew Shiels, S.G.W. Archibald,

24 "The Club," *The Novascotian*, 4 February 1830.

25 J. Murray Beck, *Joseph Howe: Conservative Reformer: 1804-1848* (Kingston and Montreal, 1982), I, p. 66.

Beamish Murdoch, T.B. Akins, Robert Cooney, and Jotham Blanchard[26] with the Club and has suggested that these people contributed in varying degrees to the development of character, dialect, and narrative (for example, there are interesting comparisons between the Scots-Canadian dialect poet, Andrew Shiels, born in Roxboroughshire, and the Club's literary original, Mr. Merlin, born on the banks of the Yarrow). However, the sustained vitality of the series clearly emanated from five central Club characters, one of whom was Mr. Editor (Joseph Howe) himself. For the other four figures, there are less clearly defined parallels, although an examination of the remaining names attributed to the Club papers does suggest certain patterns of association and characterization. Thus, the sardonic, learned Dr. Febres in the series ("our Diogenes, our Swift, our Voltaire")[27] bears many resemblances to Halifax's witty and well-spoken friend of literature, Dr. William Grigor, a Scot from Elgin who was noted for his "fine colloquial powers" and "well read, thoughtful" mind.[28] As a stock Club character, the physician provided a sharp contrast to the somewhat ethereal Barrington, a lovesick young man constantly personified in the series as a bad versifier and hopeless romantic. A poet and lawyer, as was Howe's lifelong friend, Laurence O'Connor Doyle, Barrington may well have emerged from Club sessions that were not dissimilar to the nights Howe nostalgically recalled years later:

---

26   Andrew Shiels ("Albyn") was a Scottish-born blacksmith and poet who lived in Dartmouth. A prolific writer of verse, he often contributed poetry to *The Novascotian*. S.G.W. Archibald was born in Truro, N.S., in 1777 and had a distinguished career as a lawyer, M.L.A. for Halifax County and later Colchester County, Speaker of the House of Assembly (1825-40), and a member of the Executive Council. He was known for his wit and in mid-career published clever letters in *The Acadian Recorder* under such pseudonyms as "Perigrinus" and "Anthony Doodledoo." Beamish Murdoch was a lawyer and historian who edited *The Acadian Magazine* in 1826-27. He was an M.L.A. for Halifax Township from 1826 to 1830 but is best known for his three-volume *History of Nova Scotia* (1865-67). T.B. Akins was a lawyer and historian who is credited with preserving many of Nova Scotia's earliest books and documents. He assisted both Thomas Chandler Haliburton and Beamish Murdoch in the preparation of their histories. Made Commissioner of Records in 1857, Akins was known for his *History of Halifax* (1847; 1895). Robert Cooney was an Irish-born Methodist clergyman from New Brunswick who published *A Compendious History of the Northern Part of the Province of New Brunswick* with Howe in 1832. He served in the ministry throughout North America and died in Toronto in 1870. Jotham Blanchard was educated at Pictou Academy and was editor and founder of *The Colonial Patriot* (Pictou) from 1827 to 1833. He spent part of 1828 in Halifax but probably did not contribute to "The Club" at that time, given Howe's rather antagonistic response to him (see Beck, *Joseph Howe*, I, pp. 48-52). By 1830, when Blanchard became M.L.A. for Halifax County, relations with Howe had improved, and he may have contributed to "The Club" at this time.

27   "The Club," *The Novascotian*, 8 May 1828.

28   "The Late Dr. Grigor," *The Halifax Sun*, 17 November 1857.

Mr Doyle and I commenced life together, and have a thousand personal social ties, which neither can readily forget. Many of the gayest and instructive [*sic*] of our days and nights were spent together. We spent them not in sport or wine, but in search of deep philosophy, wit, eloquence and poesy, arts which I loved, for they, my friend, were thine.

I might say...that Mr. Doyle is the only man I ever knew who had not an enemy; whose humor never flagged; whose wit never wounded; who, by common consent was everywhere welcome, and who, if immortality could be conferred by universal suffrage, everybody would vote that he would enliven every scene of festivity down to the end of time. I am quite sure if he lived so long the last trump would drown the ring of merry voices over his last jest.[29]

Renowned as he was for this character and for his clever turns of phrase, Doyle may well have contributed as much to the punning dimension of the Club selections as did the more frequently cited Thomas Chandler Haliburton.[30] Certainly, it is Howe's memory of Doyle that complements popular perceptions of the Club and contributes to the image of the Howe coterie as a clever and eloquent gathering of wits.

In Major Metheglin, the crusty old veteran of the Peninsular campaigns and the Battle of Waterloo, there are many resemblances to Captain (later, Sir) John Kinkaid, an officer from Wellington's Peninsular campaigns who was stationed in Halifax with the 95th Regiment of Rifles during most of the Club series. Always the emotional and dramatic focus of the Club in its early years, the Major has finished his "Recollections of the Peninsula" coincident with Kinkaid's completing his *Adventures in the Rifle Brigade, in the Peninsula, France and the Netherlands*, published in London in 1830. The sudden removal of the Major from the sketches in January 1830 may have set the stage for Kinkaid's return to Great Britain and his subsequent resignation from the army, a development disguised in the Club by the story that the Major was away in London attending to the business of the King. With the Major's departure, however, the Club began to lose an important unifying focus, for the bluff old "champion and fire-eater"[31] was the lifeblood of the group ("Oh! for half an hour of the Major and his criticisms," says the Doctor

---

29 George Mullane, "A Sketch of Laurence O'Connor Doyle, A Member of the House of Assembly in the Thirties and Forties," *Collections of the Nova Scotia Historical Society*, XVII (1913), p. 169.

30 For a reference to Haliburtons' punning abilities, see V.L.O. Chittick, *Thomas Chandler Haliburton: A Study in Provincial Toryism* (New York, 1924), pp. 121-22.

31 "The Club," *The Novascotian*, 21 January 1830.

mournfully on 14 May 1830).[32] Soon recognizing that the loss of the Major was undermining the dramatic unity of the sketches, the Club animateurs decided to re-introduce his character in September 1830. However, the role he assumed in the later sketches was more cautious and didactic than dramatic, and there is every suggestion in the anti-climactic nature of the Major's character in the last year of the Club that no writer of Kinkaid's literary strength could be found to develop the military background and heartiness necessary to maintain the consistency of the Major's character. It is significant that when the Club series finally ended in October 1831, the character of the Major had so diminished in importance that Mr Merlin, not the Major, was given the task of delivering the final farewell.

Although much has been written about Thomas Chandler Haliburton, the remaining member of the original Club group, little has been said about his contribution to the Club series. Here, as is the case with a number of other members of the group, little documentation about the author's literary activities in the 1820s survives. However, Haliburton's involvement with the Club circle was a natural development in a series of literary associations and influences stretching from his college years in Windsor to the 1826-29 period when he was a Member of the House of Assembly for Annapolis and a member of the Club. Throughout those years, he had always enjoyed friendships with literarily inclined people — first with such fellow students at King's as the Blisses and the Parkers of New Brunswick[33] and later with more established figures like the Honourable Peleg Wiswall of Digby. Describing "want of society"[34] in Annapolis as the initial catalyst for his turning to writing, Haliburton had published *A General Description of Nova Scotia* by the time he was only 27 and had continued to work on his more major *An Historical and Statistical Account of Nova Scotia* throughout the mid and late 1820s. His desire to achieve success as a writer had emerged not only in his determination to produce a provincial history even in the midst of a burgeoning legal and political career, but also in his correspondence on the topic with a friend and adviser like Peleg Wiswall:

32   *Ibid.*, 14 May 1830.

33   Robert and Neville Parker of Saint John were sons of Loyalists and attended King's while Haliburton was a student there. Both became Supreme Court Judges before becoming Chief Justice (Robert) and Master of the Rolls (Neville) in New Brunswick. Both were literarily inclined and published in *The Acadian Magazine* under the pseudonyms "Atticus" (Robert) and "Cecil" (Neville). Henry Bliss and William Bliss of Saint John were other classmates and friends of Haliburton and the Parker brothers. A lawyer with a literary bent, Henry Bliss was later to live in England and publish his verse and drama there under the pseudonym Nicholas Thirning Moile. The Bliss Letters in the Public Archives of Nova Scotia reveal a lively Halifax social circle which includes references to Haliburton and his family.

34   Tho. C. Haliburton to "Dear Sir" [Peleg Wiswall], 31 December 1823, Wiswall Collection, MG 1, vol. 979, Folder 1, PANS.

Whoever is known in this province as the author of any publication must consider that he has voluntarily brought himself to the Stake to be baited, by the empty barking of some and the stings and bites of others. If he is not known and his work attains to mediocrity it will not be censured for fear that it should be the work of some established character, nor praised for fear that applause should fall upon an unknown, whom the generality of wits if they had not considered as their inferior are at all events not disposed to place higher than on an exact level with themselves. The Price of Printing, too, at Halifax, is beyond all reason and failure would be ruin. My intention was to go on progressively but steadily till I had finished the entire work, when I should send a correct Copy to my friend Francklin in London and desire him to sell it to a bookseller for the best price he could obtain if he could not sell it to give it to the printer if he would publish it at his own cost, and if he could not dispose of it to light his pipe with it. For I am not one who would rebel at the decision of the Booksellers and say "Sdeath I'll print it and shame the fools." I think their judgement infallible. They have administered so long to the literary appetite of the Public that they understand as it were by instinct what will be palatable and what will be removed from the table untouched. Everything however which has America for its Subject, (how dull or absurd soever it may be) is read in England with avidity, and I am not altogether without hopes of being able to dispose of my labours in some way or other.[35]

Such sentiments suggest just how self-conscious about writing Haliburton had become by 1824 and may explain the continuing activity ("progressively but steadily") and anonymity which marked his pursuit of his writing ventures once he had moved into Halifax literary circles in the late 1820s. Identified by Archibald MacMechan as part of *The Acadian Magazine* coterie of Beamish Murdoch, James Foreman, and J. Scott Tremaine,[36] Haliburton in fact made no known contributions to the periodical in the 1826 to 1828 period. With its engraving of Windsor, its sense of historical continuity, its pride in Annapolis Royal and Windsor, and its vision of progress, the poem "Western Scenes" published in the journal in January 1827 is highly reminiscent of Haliburton's interests and philosophy. However, the poem

---

35   Tho. C. Haliburton to "Dear Sir" [Peleg Wiswall], 7 January 1824, *ibid.*

36   Archibald MacMechan, "Thomas Haliburton," MacMechan Papers, Ms. 2/82/F29, p. 3, Dalhousie University Archives.

remains anonymous in origin,[37] and it is therefore to the Club sketches of 1828 and 1829 that one must turn for the first manifestations of Haliburton's creative talents.

Haliburton's contribution to the Club was two-fold: first, as a dramatic, literal figure taking part in the Club exchanges, and, second, as a force behind the scenes helping to shape the humour and characterization of the series. As a dramatic character, he brings a note of authenticity to the fictional conversations by appearing under his own name and by openly sharing his mockery of the House of Assembly with the Club members. What strikes the reader immediately is that there is very little distinction between the fictional persona of Thomas Chandler Haliburton in the Club sequences and the public man known in the House and the courts for his clever turns of phrase and reductive humour. Describing Haliburton's performance on the floor of the Legislature in 1829, *The Acadian Recorder* frequently refers to his "witticisms" or his "usual flow of wit,"[38] and Judge J.A. Stewart notes in a letter to Peleg Wiswall in the autumn of 1829 that Haliburton's appointment to the bench in Windsor is receiving support from his fellow legislators merely because they wish to rid themselves of his thorny, quick-tongued presence in the House:

> The Lawyers [in the house], say what they will, are to a man, from the Speaker, downward, rejoiced to have him out of their way — independent of his being on the road to the Chair, he was troublesome to many individual members who were afraid of his wit and his sarcasm, and they must feel happy that he cannot come again among them. — Some think that the Governor appointed him to the office to get rid of him, and others think that My Old Friend the Treasurer, as well as the Attorney-General, and even the good Bishop, will not lament the appointment *at heart*.[39]

That this public persona was carried into the fictional presentation of Haliburton in the Club papers is clear from the inquisition sketch of 1829 when the Club is attempting to investigate the background of John Alexander Barry's expulsion from the House of Assembly and the cause of the riot that

---

37 For a discussion of "Western Scenes" see Gwendolyn Davies, "A Literary Study of Selected Periodicals From Maritime Canada: 1789-1872", Ph.D. thesis, York University, 1979, pp. 64-73. See also Tom Vincent, *"The Acadian Magazine"* in William Toye, ed., *The Oxford Companion to Canadian Literature* (Toronto, 1983), p. 4.

38 "Provincial Parliament, Nova Scotia," *The Acadian Recorder*, 14 March 1829.

39 J.A. Stewart to Peleg Wiswall, 5 October 1829, Wiswall Collection, MG 1, Vol. 980, p. 40. PANS.

ensued.[40] Relishing wit as they do, the Club members are looking forward to Haliburton's visit because of his reputation for saying "some devilish good things"[41] on the floor of the House. Thus, the Club devotees treat Haliburton with genuine affection when he comes before them to answer their queries about his behaviour in the incident and the reasons why he voted against the member from Shelburne. As the exchange continues, Haliburton's comments on Barry's conduct reflect the pattern of ironic reduction so typical of both the Club humour and of some of the later Sam Slick sketches and illustrate how effective a well-developed character can be in focusing the satiric thrust of a sketch. Questioned by the Major, the chief officer of the inquisition, Haliburton first responds to inquiries about Barry by tossing off a round of puns on one's "bolting" and being bolted in, and then goes on to sum up Barry's appeal to a man of irony like himself:

> I'll tell you my opinion of it, but first, I must say, this is a noble cigar,what a flavour it has. I always get my talking tacks aboard when I get a cigar in my mouth...I was sorry to have to vote against him, I shall miss him terribly he was such a good subject for ridicule. I used to like to spear him, for it never hurt his feelings, as he could not understand a joke.[42]

In Haliburton's comment, "I shall miss him terribly...he was such a good subject for ridicule," there is an anticipation of Sam Slick's later observation, "When reason fails to convince, there's nothing left but ridicule."[43] While this philosophy could be said to sum up not only Sam's *raison d'être* but also the Club's, it also supports the image of Haliburton that emerges when life meets art. Clever at repartee before the Club members and fast on his feet before the House, there is no inconsistency between the man who defends ridicule as a therapeutic device on the floor of the Assembly and the man who a few years later will try to stir his countrymen to action through the imaginative parries and thrusts of his provocateur, Sam Slick. The doctor in the Club objects to this image, remarking somewhat dourly after Haliburton's appearance before the mock-tribunal that "the making of laws is a serious business — and smiles cannot assist the despatch of important business."[44]

---

40 For a description of the Barry affair, see Beck, *Joseph Howe*, I, pp. 58-64, and George Cox, "John Alexander Barry and His Times," *Collections of the Nova Scotia Historical Society* , 28 (1949), pp. 133-46.

41 "The Club," *The Novascotian*, 5 June 1828.

42 *Ibid.*, 21 May 1829.

43 [Thomas Chandler Haliburton], *The Clockmaker; Or, The Sayings and Doings of Samuel Slick, of Slickville* (Halifax, 1836), p. 69.

44 "The Club," *The Novascotian*, 21 May 1829.

However, it is consistent with the dialectical nature of the Club that the Major leaps to Haliburton's defence here, pointing out the fine distinction between a clever turn of mind and an insightful approach to legislation. His summation — "No, Sir, you may depend upon this...the very agility of mind so to speak, which is necessary to the making of a good joke, is of service in making a good law"[45] — is almost an affirmation of the Club's role and responsibility as much as it is a defence of Haliburton. In the eyes of the Major, wit is always to be an able weapon in legislating the direction of fools.

Although the character of Thomas Chandler Haliburton in the Club sequences bore a resemblance to the public man, Haliday, the fictional figure whom he inspired, is less visibly characteristic. In Haliday, the vivacious and fair-minded young lawyer, one has a typical Club member — a lover of his glass, a capable punster, an admirer of justice, and a genuine party-goer and patriot:

> One Toast more, before the Music. Brew again, my hearties, — a Toast which shall find reverberation in every sound heart within the three Provinces. Here is a bumper to "the Novascotian" — may its roots continue to sink deeper in our soil and its leaves still spread their umbrageous and kindly influence over a free and happy people.[46]

What is particularly interesting about the Haliday figure, however, is the role he plays in the sketches as a catalyst to the Major, for just as the Squire in the Clockmaker series is later to act as a foil for Sam Slick by asking questions that stimulate Sam's responses, so, here, Haliday's queries usually initiate a disquisition from the main spokesman of the Club, the Major:

> Haliday: Pray what do you call the essentials of a young ladies' education; you are so original in your notions, I should like to hear you on that subject.
> Major: I call the knowledge of her duty to God, to her parents, and society, an essential....[47]
> or:
> Haliday: But Major, how comes it, you are up in arms for his Majesty's customs? Do you expect Jeffery to resign in your favour as colonial Aide-de Camp?
> Major Sir, you trifle, no Sir; I perceive now....[48]

---

45 *Ibid.*

46 "Grand Pantomime," *ibid.*, 13 January 1830.

47 "The Club," *ibid.*, 5 February 1829. This sketch has the initials T.C.H. written beside it on the Canadian Library Association microfilm of *The Novascotian*.

48 *Ibid.*, 9 February 1829.

It is impossible to know the extent of Haliburton's involvement in writing scenarios like these in the Club papers, but in the surviving *Novascotian* sketch with "T.C.H." written beside it, there are further illustrations of this same stimulus-response technique. Certainly, the success of the pattern in the Club sketches must have provided Haliburton with a salutary example of the effectiveness of counterpointing in developing the tension and narrative pace of a short newspaper piece. While the technique is less obvious in the Club sketches than in the later Clockmaker series because of the way in which it becomes integrated into the conversations of other Club members, the same stimulus-response mechanisms function in both series to effect a dramatic focus often lacking in conversational exchanges of this kind. Intermittent as Haliburton's association with the Club group was to become by the middle of 1829, it seems very probable that his involvement with Howe's series did much to facilitate the development of the strongly contrasted characters, vital language, and counterpointing dialogue which were to be part of his success in developing the satirical thrust of the 1835 Sam Slick sketches.

The Haliday-Haliburton figure disappears from the Club in December 1830, dying, appropriately enough, from choking on a pun. "I have to deplore the loss of one of the most distinguished members of the Club — ," notes the Major forlornly: "Haliday, the gay, the witty, the philosophic Haliday, expired in a fit of laughter at our last best pun."[49] His demise followed Haliburton's removal from Halifax to a Judgeship in Windsor by nearly a year, and during that time eleven Haliday sketches had appeared in the newspaper. It is entirely possible that Haliburton continued to contribute to the Club during that period, for transportation between Windsor and Halifax was fast and frequent by colonial standards. However, it is more likely that members of the group sustained the Haliday fiction by working with established conventions. That they were genuinely concerned about the loss of such an ebullient and unifying character from the sketches is clear from their attempts to keep his memory alive even after he had been officially pronounced dead, and for this reason the authors of the Club brought the literal ghost of Haliday back a number of times during 1830-31 to partake of the festivities of his former comrades and to bring a touch of his old gaiety and charm to the proceedings:

> (Here there is a sudden noise as of a rush of wind, through the keyhole a thin vapour issues, dilates, grows more perceptible to the eye, and gradually assumes the attitude and form of Haliday.)
> Doctor — The spirit of our departed friend; Frank, my dear fellow, incarnate or disembodied, thou art welcome; and whatever "air from

---

49 *Ibid.*, 1 December 1830.

Heaven" you may bring, you know we will never shrink from the *draught*.

Major — Here is to you, Frank; nothing like a "communion of spirits". You can crack a bottle yet, can you not?

Haliday — Come, Doctor, I'll give you a subject for discussion....[50]

However, just as suddenly as the Haliday character reappeared and disappeared from the Club gatherings, so after three years of publication, the sketches themselves suddenly ceased without warning on 12 October 1831. Characteristically enough, the announcement was made in one of the many drinking songs which dot the text and stress the fellowship of the group. And it is that spirit of conviviality — not the reasons for the Club's dispersal — that dominates Mr. Merlin's presentation in this last appearance: "Farewell, once again, to each man of the Club,/ And, oh! many a laugh I shall have/ When I think of the pun, and the joke and the rub,/ That you all so good humouredly gave."[51]

However, in spite of the fact that no explanations were given for the termination of the Club series, a close reading of the sketches in the last year of their existence may provide some insights into the decision of Howe and his colleagues to end the sequence while it was still popular and still respected. Although it had continued to tackle matters of social relevance to Nova Scotia in 1830-31, it had nonetheless lost much of the original spontaneity with which it had treated both dialogue and subject matter. The departure of such experienced and knowledgeable writers as Captain Kincaid and Thomas Chandler Haliburton could never be rectified, even with the addition of new authors, and it was only in the conception of the Mr. Merlin figure that Howe was able to recapture some of the vitality and originality that had made the Major a keystone in the organization and dramatic unity of the series. Moreover, by 1831, only Howe, Grigor, and Doyle remained from the original group, and it is quite possible that they were finding it increasingly difficult to sustain the quality and frequency of the Club papers as their own careers gathered momentum and as their political interests led them inexorably closer to the hustings and election to the House of Assembly.

Finally, it could be argued that the Club papers came to an end when they did because they had accomplished what they could in ridiculing the follies and inequities of the society around them, and had exhausted their uniqueness as part of the on-going process of satirical writing which had characterized Nova Scotian literary life and Halifax newspapers throughout the decade of the 1820s. However, as a successor to satirical writers like Thomas McCulloch, T.S.B., Peregrinus, and Censor, the Club represents an important

---

50   *Ibid.*, 10 February 1831.

51   "Merlin's Farewell To The Club," *ibid.*, 12 October 1831.

stage in the developing pattern of Nova Scotian satire that was to culminate in the birth of Sam Slick in 1835. More outward-looking and more diversified in their development of personae than McCulloch's letters, and more spontaneous and erudite than any Nova Scotian satire to this time, the Club sketches anticipated the social thrust, vivid language, and dramatic qualities that were to make the Sam Slick narratives so memorable. Moreover, it can be argued that it is with the Club that Thomas Chandler Haliburton learned the effectiveness of many of the techniques (and addressed many of the subjects) that were to be refined in the "Recollections of Nova Scotia" (*The Clockmaker*) just a few years later. To meet the conversational demands of the Club sessions, Haliburton and the other writers in the series gained practical experience in learning how to write colloquially, in discovering how to develop a personal and intimate relationship with the reader, and in recognizing the possibilities that dialect afforded them in developing humorous and satirical effects. All this practical background Haliburton undoubtedly found useful when he turned to the shaping of Sam Slick, partly a child of the Yankee and Western dialect traditions of America, but also a character as bumptious and as opinionated in his own way as Mr. Merlin or Major Metheglin in the Club.

Howe, Haliburton, and company have left few recollections of the Club beyond the published sketches, but in after years they always spoke of the friendships and the conversations of the late 1820s with great affection and nostalgia. In the demand to meet a newspaper deadline — and in the need to create vivid, fictional characters as the interpreters and messengers of their opinions — they also learned to write satire quickly and well. Literary history has forgotten the role that the Club papers played in honing their reforming and creative talents, but in the surviving pages of *The Novascotian*, there are glimpses of their academy — those festive nights in the Club Room, communing over the fellowship of the bowl:

The Meeting of the Club

Oh! There's not in this wide world so snug a retreat
As the little back room where the merry Club meet;
Oh! the last ray of feeling and life shall depart,
Ere the joys of that conclave shall fade from my heart.

Oh! it is not that Nature has spread o'er the scene
Her fairest Havanahs, and choicest Poteen;
Oh! it is not the wine cup we frequently fill,
Oh! no, it is something more exquisite still.

'Tis the converse of friends whom our bosoms hold dear —
The jokes which we crack, and the songs that we hear:
And which show how the charms of the Table improve
When by wit they're reflected from spirits we love.[52]

---

52 "Grand Pantomime," *ibid.*, 13 January 1830.

Note: For further discussion of the Club Papers, see Carrie MacMillan, "Colonial Gleanings: 'The Club' Papers (1828-31)," *Essays on Canadian Writing*, 31 (Summer 1985), pp. 51-64.

William Charles M'Kinnon:
Cape Breton's Sir Walter Scott

From the publication of *Waverley* in 1814 to the conclusion of the *Tales of My Landlord* in 1832, the novels of Sir Walter Scott enjoyed a popularity in North America unrivalled by that of any other British writer.[1] With their sense of a chivalric code, their intriguing villain-heroes, their tribute to the common man, and their almost epic-like interpretation of history, Scott's novels brought an energy and originality to fiction that seemed highly refreshing after the self-conscious moral tales of the eighteenth century. "The appearance of a new novel from his pen caused a greater sensation in the United States than did some of the battles of Napoleon...," noted Samuel Goodrich. "Everybody read these works; everybody — the refined and the simple — shared in the delightful trances which seemed to transport them to remote ages and distant climes, and made them live and breathe in the presence of the stern Covenanters of Scotland, the gallant bowmen of Sherwood Forest, or even the Crusaders in Palestine."[2]

That Scott was as popular in Nova Scotia as he was in the United States is clear from letters, articles, and advertisements emanating from the province in the nineteenth century. Scott novels were usually reviewed in Halifax newspapers only months after appearing in Great Britain,[3] and booksellers lost little time in importing the latest work from the master's pen. Newspapers and periodicals allowed subscribers to read recent serializations of Scott from abroad,[4] and personal correspondence offered family and friends the opportunity to discuss the intricacies of his characterizations and plots. Writing to Henry Bliss in Fredericton in 1816, Sarah Ann Anderson was typical of many Nova Scotians in wanting to engage a sympathetic fellow reader in an analysis of a recent novel by "The Great Unknown."[5]

---

1   James D. Hart, *The Popular Book, A History of America's Literary Taste* (Berkeley and Los Angeles, 1963), p. 73.

2   *Ibid.*, p. 74.

3   For example, see *The Nova-Scotia Royal Gazette*, 14 June 1826. *Woodstock* had appeared in London in May 1826 and a review was published in Halifax in June.

4   For an example, see excerpts from *The Fortunes of Nigel, Acadian Recorder*, 3-10 August 1822. In addition to being available through conventional avenues, Scott could occasionally be bought when a private library was being dispersed. For example, an advertisement appearing in the Halifax *Weekly Chronicle* on 21 December 1821 offered to sell several of Mr. B. O'Meara's books, including *Ivanhoe* and *The Monastery*.

5   Scott's identity as a novelist was suspected for a number of years before he publicly confessed authorship in 1827. Until then, the mystery surrounding the authorship of the *Waverley* novels led to their being credited to "The Great Unknown" and "The Wizard of the North."

"You are charmed with my friend Meg," she noted, after receiving Bliss's letter on *Guy Mannering*, "and let me tell you, nothing pleased me more than to read her praises, for I think I never met a fictitious character in whom I took so lively an interest." On the whole, however, she and Mr. Bliss differed in their assessment of the author's protagonists. Bliss was critical of Scott's dominie because he was too much an "original" to be believable. She defended such a character portrayal, seeming to find the novelist's unorthodox figures the most interesting. The "wild...forcible" language of the Meg sections and the "creatures of imagination" were to her Scott's strength. Her critical interpretations were astute and suggest a keener understanding of Scott's appeal to the general public than is implied in Bliss's more mundane responses. Nevertheless, both correspondents represent the tremendous interest in Scott that existed in their society in the first half of the nineteenth century. Gathered around the fire in family groups and reading societies, Nova Scotians like Sarah Ann Anderson heard Scott read aloud in nightly installments and for months afterwards found the writer's romances of the past a popular subject in conversation and correspondence.[6]

Given the popularity and availability of the Waverley novels in Nova Scotia, it is not surprising that a literary generation grew up in the province reflecting Scott's influence and interests. Young writers of the 1840s and 1850s like Douglas Huyghue, Mary Jane Katzmann, James DeMille and William Charles M'Kinnon often turned to historical themes in their prose and poetry and tried to articulate for Maritimers the sense of heritage and place that Scott had conveyed in his nation's literature. Of this group, William Charles M'Kinnon of North Sydney was for a short time the most active, publishing six historical romances, a collection of historical verse, and a body of periodical poetry and prose between 1844 and 1852. Like the young James DeMille, he tried to extend his literary career beyond Nova Scotia into Boston, and in the suitably-named *Waverley Magazine* found an outlet for his Scott-inspired tales of Cape Breton and the past.

William Charles M'Kinnon's references to Sir Walter Scott, Bulwer-Lytton, Captain Marryat, and James Fenimore Cooper reveal the inspiration behind much of his historical fiction, but without question M'Kinnon's interest in the past was also generated by the active participation of his own family in some of the major historical events of eighteenth and nineteenth-

---

6   Sarah Ann Anderson to Henry Bliss, Bliss Papers, MG 1, vol. 1604, 5 August 1816, Public Archives of Nova Scotia (PANS). I wish to express my appreciation to the following people for assisting me in my research for this paper: the staff of the Public Archives of Nova Scotia; the Reverend Neil MacLeod, Archivist, Pine Hill Divinity Hall; Dr. Robert Morgan, Director, the Beaton Institute of Cape Breton Studies; the Boston Public Library; and Mrs. Beryl Davis, Glace Bay, Nova Scotia. In her letter to Henry Bliss, Sarah Ann Anderson says that "the Chief" [Chief Justice Henry Blowers] had read *Guy Mannering* to the family some months before. Miss Anderson was a ward of Sampson Blowers.

century America. His great-grandfather, Thomas Hutchins, had been the first geographer-general of the United States and had enjoyed the support of the American statesman and scholar, Benjamin Franklin. A former British officer who had been imprisoned in London during the American Revolution because of suspected communications with Franklin in Paris, Hutchins had returned to America in 1780 to fight for the revolutionary cause.[7] While he remained in the United States as an honoured scholar and citizen after the War of Independence, his son-in-law, Captain William M'Kinnon, had removed to Cape Breton as a Loyalist refugee in December, 1792. A captain with the Provincials during the war, M'Kinnon described himself on his arrival in Sydney as "robbed of his all by the enemys of his country."[8] After difficulties over M'Kinnon's property claims had been resolved,[9] he settled into Cape Breton life as a vestryman in St. George's Anglican Church, a Registrar of Deeds, a member of the Executive Council, and the Provincial Secretary of Cape Breton. When he died in 1811 from the effects of a wound received on board the "Bristol" at Sullivan's Island during the War of Independence, he was given a full military funeral in Sydney as a captain in the British Army. With a sense of pageantry befitting a Walter Scott novel, the 104th Regiment marched through the streets of the town "in breeches and white stockings and with drums muffled with crepe, and fifes playing the dead March of 'Rosslyn Castle,' and a farewell salute of three volleys was fired over his grave."[10]

William Charles M'Kinnon's personal contact with history extended into his father's generation, for John M'Kinnon joined the 104th Regiment of Line while still under 20. In the War of 1812, Lieutenant M'Kinnon was wounded while serving under Sir Gordon Drummond in the Canadas and in 1817 went on half-pay. For the next 30 years he took an active part in Cape Breton life as a magistrate and as a Lieutenant-Colonel commanding a battalion of militia. However, according to his widow, Catherine MacDonald M'Kinnon, her husband was so debilitated by his wounds that he eventually had to mortgage and sell his farm in order to educate and raise their eight

---

7   For a capsule summary of Thomas Hutchins' life, see *The National Cyclopaedia of American Biography*, IX (Ann Arbor, 1967), p. 267. Margaret Hutchins M'Kinnon, wife of William M'Kinnon, died at Kill Marie near Sydney on 30 January 1840. I am grateful to Mrs. Beryl Davis for drawing my attention to Margaret M'Kinnon's obituary in *The Novascotian* on 20 February 1840.

8   See Petition of William M'Kinnon, Esquire, to His Honor Lieutenant General Despard, MG 1, D25, Beaton Institute Archives, Sydney; also see Micro. Box 27, and petition for land grant in 1793, Muggah Papers, MG 12, 68/B1.

9   R. Brown, *A History of the Island of Cape Breton* (London, 1869), pp. 412-13.

10   J.G. MacKinnon, *Old Sydney* (Sydney, 1918), p. 95.

children.[11] What Catherine M'Kinnon did not report to Lord Mulgrave in 1863 when she applied for a military pension was that her husband had also been reduced to selling patent medicines in an effort to support his family. It is as the purveyor of the British College of Health's "Morison's Pills" that John M'Kinnon was best known locally. During his years as an agent, he tried to set up sub-agencies throughout Cape Breton, at one point petitioning the Provincial Legislature to admit Morison's medicines into Nova Scotia free of duty.[12] He also advertised himself as the agent for Du Barry's Revalenta Food,[13] and during his son's publishing days in North Sydney, seems to have operated a stationery business in the offices of both *The Cape-Breton Spectator* and *The Times*.[14]

Born on 19 April 1828, William Charles M'Kinnon was the eldest of Lieutenant John M'Kinnon's children. It is interesting to speculate on the influences that encouraged the young M'Kinnon to write, for with the exception of a few occasional poets, no English-speaking author of his literary aspirations had yet emerged from the Sydney area by the middle of the 1840s. If M'Kinnon's fictional description of the North Sydney of his boyhood is any indication, the port area was exotic enough an environment to excite the imagination of any literarily-inclined youth. It was a place of "few buildings," "stir and bustle," and a "harbour...crowded with vessels of all sizes and of all nations."[15] The burgeoning coal industry was converting the quiet rural area into a growing port centre, and at the dockside, one could find "the little street running parallel with the water... filled with a busy crowd:"

> The full-faced, good humored, but highly gullible Englishman — the sallow, sharp featured American — the Newfoundlander in his Pea-jacket and Southwester — the Frenchman from St. Pierre — the native Cape Breton sailor, aping, by his slang oaths, his belt, bowie knife, et cetera, the appearance of the Yankee — the dust stained miner — the colonist, with his cart of produce — the Backlander, speaking a mixture

11   "The Memorial of Catherine McKinnon" to "His Excellency The Right Honorable Earl of Mulgrave," RG 5, Series "GP", Misc. "A", vol. 4, No. 177, PANS.

12   In January 1846, Mr. J.B. Uniacke presented the petition of John M'Kinnon and several hundred others asking to have Morison's Pills introduced duty-free. The petition provoked much hilarity in the legislature according to the Halifax *Morning Post* on 19 January 1846 and to the Sydney *Spirit of the Times* on 28 January 1846. The episode inspired Mordecai Levi to write a poem for the *Morning Post* on 27 January 1846 entitled "Important testimonial Respecting Morison's Pills." Typical advertisements for John M'Kinnon's franchise as an agent for the British College of Health's Medicines can be found in *The Cape-Breton Spectator*, 14 August and 13 November 1847.

13   See *The Cape-Breton News*, 7 June 1851.

14   See *The Cape-Breton Spectator*, 18 December 1847.

15   W.C. M'Kinnon, *The Midnight Murder. A Legend of Cape Breton*, in *The Waverley Magazine*, 16 November 1850.

of broken English and Gaelic — the Coaster, swearing at the delay in not being allowed to load, as he spit forth his tobacco juice more energetically as he contemplated the idea — the embryo merchant prince retailing liquor at an advance of two hundred per cent — the woolly-pated negro, shivering with the cold — the loafer, with a pipe in his mouth and his hands in his pockets, looking as unconcerned as if he had nothing to win or lose in the great Battle of Life — all united in making the scene one of unparalleled confusion.[16]

If the dockside environment of North Sydney were this active in 1833 when the notorious Flahaven murder took place in the town,[17] it is not surprising that M'Kinnon retained a vivid enough memory of the scene to incorporate it into his 1850 fictionalization of the event, *The Midnight Murder. A Legend of Cape Breton*.[18] However, much of his childhood seems to have been spent on his father's rural acreage at Leitche's Creek, and surviving records for the Northside North West Arm schoolhouse where Lieutenant John M'Kinnon was one of the trustees indicate that William Charles M'Kinnon spent the year 1839 with 41 other scholars engaged in studies of "reading, writing, and arithmetic."[19] While this school was classified as a "first class" institution,[20] it seems likely that parental guidance, not the rural schoolroom, directed and shaped the author's literary tastes.[21] No record of the family library exists, but it is known that Beattie's *Scotland Illustrated,* Lady Prévost's *Defence of Sir George Prévost's Administration* and Bink's *Theological Dictionary* were among the books in the M'Kinnon home.[22] As well, William Charles M'Kinnon's familiarity with the Bible[23] and his deep interest in ornithology, navigation, astronomy, and

---

16   *Ibid.*

17   For an account of the murder, see MacKinnon, *Old Sydney*, pp. 58-62.

18   *The Midnight Murder. A Legend of Cape Breton* appeared first in *The Commercial Herald* of Sydney on 23 March 1850. It subsequently appeared in *The Waverley Magazine* of Boston on 16 November 1850.

19   School Return, Northside North West Arm, RG 14, Vols. 5-6, no. 22, PANS.

20   *Ibid.*; the teacher was Thomas Hyde. For an interesting account of the state of the schools in the Sydney area in 1841 during William Charles M'Kinnon's childhood, see the "Report of School Commissions, County of Cape Breton, RG 14, Vols. 5-6, no. 23, PANS.

21   G.O. Heustis, "Memorials of the Late Rev. W.C. M'Kinnon," *Provincial Wesleyan*, 18 June 1862.

22   John M'Kinnon had "30 numbers" of Dr. Beattie's "Scotland Illustrated" which he advertised as "nearly new" in *The Cape-Breton Spectator*, 20 October 1847. Three years later, he asked that persons borrowing his *Bink's Theological Dictionary* and *Lady Prévost's Defence of Sir George Prévost's Administration to Canada, during the Last American War* send his books home without delay. This appeared in *The Commercial Herald*, 23 March 1850.

23   Heustis, "Memorials," p. 2.

composition,[24] all suggest a domestic environment conducive to study and intellectual pursuit.

William Charles M'Kinnon's first major literary work, *The Battle of the Nile*, reveals a confident familiarity with classical history and the masters of English poetry. Containing several poems — "The Steep of Fame," "Life," "An Elegy To the Shade of Thomas Campbell, L.C.D." and "The Battle of the Nile" — the book is important in articulating M'Kinnon's early fascination with "the imaginative breathings of Romance." "The reader's good sense...will pardon these little flights, in the following pages," notes the author: "If seen in prose," such "imaginative breathings of Romance" would "call forth ridicule."[25] However, appearing under the guise of poetry, such romantic expressions are only an illustration of the fact that "the poet is compelled to write beyond what he intends."[26]

A 39 page account of Napoleon's defeat by Nelson in Egypt, the title poem suggests the almost epic-like importance of Britain's victory over the French by putting it in the context of great battles from the time of Hector, the Ptolemies, and Hannibal. Having established a sense of history and continuum in the poem, M'Kinnon then employs the next three cantos to sketch in the background and reputation of his two protagonists, Napoleon and Nelson. Inevitably, the poem moves through progressive stages or arguments, culminating in the dramatic sea confrontation of the two leaders. A quick and decisive dénouement follows, proclaiming that "England once more is sovereign of the main/ Where Nelson's mighty arm her rights maintain;/ His streamers wave from Nilus' slimy shore,/ To Denmark and Iberia — streaming o'er."[27]

The tone of "The Battle of the Nile" is always brisk, muscular, and confident, much in the style of the popular historical verse of Sir Walter Scott. What is striking about the poem and its companion pieces is that William Charles M'Kinnon was only sixteen years old when J.D. Kuhn published the collection in Sydney in 1844, and in their breadth of allusion and poetic control, the poems represent an extraordinary achievement for someone so young. While most of the poems give evidence of craftsmanship rather than originality, they illustrate a maturity of mind and sophistication in style that does much to explain M'Kinnon's emergence as a publisher, editor, and writer only two years later. Beginning with *The Cape-Breton Spectator* in 1846, M'Kinnon was to found and edit three newspapers over a four year period. *The Cape-Breton Spectator* (1846-48) and *The Times and Cape-Breton Spectator* (1849) emanated from North Sydney, while *The*

---

24   *Ibid.*

25   William C. M'Kinnon, *The Battle of the Nile* (Sydney, 1844), p. 3.

26   *Ibid.*

27   *Ibid.*, p. 44.

Commercial Herald (1850) operated out of Sydney. However, in a sense all three papers served the same constituency of Sydney and rural Cape Breton, and two of them appeared under mastheads linking them to the historical writers, Sir Walter Scott and Edward Bulwer-Lytton.[28]

In the late 1840s when M'Kinnon began to publish his newspapers, the Sydneys were small port towns with a social and intellectual life organized around the Scientific and Literary Society, the Mechanics' Institute, and local town bands.[29] However, Sydney's situation as a sea port meant that it suffered little time lag in receiving news and books from overseas, and the well-stocked store of John Bourinot, father of the future author and parliamentary authority, Sir John Bourinot, ensured Sydney-area residents of the most recent periodicals with their serializations of Dickens, Bulwer-Lytton, Marryat, and Cooper.[30] Patterns for the latest fashions arrived seasonally from Halifax,[31] the temperance societies organized social occasions and sponsored talks,[32] and community hospitality formed the basis

28 M'Kinnon deeply admired Scott and Bulwer-Lytton and dedicated his last novel, *St. George*, to Bulwer-Lytton. *The Cape-Breton Spectator* appeared under a Sir Walter Scott masthead, "This is my own, my native land," a sentiment which expressed the newspaper's Cape Breton leanings. The *Herald* was published under a Bulwer-Lytton masthead, "Beneath the Rule of Men Entirely Great, The Pen is Mightier than the Sword." In a sense, this quotation suggests the advocacy role M'Kinnon ascribed to newspapers.

29 There is little evidence in the newspapers of there being a theatre life in Sydney prior to the 1850s. *The Cape Breton Spectator*, 18 December 1847, mentions the stormy voyage from Sydney to Boston experienced by Rockwell's Circus Company. Whether this group performed in Sydney or merely passed through the town is unclear. On 20 May 1854 an advertisement for the Theatre Royal appeared in *The Cape Breton News*. Performed by amateurs of the 74th Regiment in the Temperance Hall, the plays of the evening included *Douglas; Or the Noble Shepherd* and *Cramond Berg; or the Days of King James the 5th of Scotland*. The evening ended with "a laughable farce, *The Haunted Inn*." For a discussion of Sydney cultural life in the 1840s, see Kenneth Donovan, "'May Learning Flourish': The Beginnings of a Cultural Awakening in Cape Breton During the 1840's," in Kenneth Donovan, ed., *The Island. New Perspectives on Cape Breton History. 1713-1990* (Fredericton and Sydney, 1990), pp. 89-112.

30 For a good example of the kind of list carried by John Bourinot in his store, see "New Books," *The Spirit of the Times*, 19 July 1842. In addition to selling recent periodicals such as *Chamber's Edinburgh Journal* and *Penny and Saturday Magazine*, Bourinot had "James's two last novels" and "Bulwer's last novel — *Zanoni*." Both G.P.R. James and Bulwer-Lytton succeeded in keeping interest in the historical novel alive. The availability of their books in Sydney reveals one of the influences shaping William Charles M'Kinnon's taste in fiction.

31 For example, see the advertisement of James Leddy, Tailor, in *The Spirit of the Times*, 19 July 1842.

32 The Temperance society in the Sydneys probably appealed to young people because it did offer entertainment. In January 1850, for example, the Archangel Division of Sydney Mines sponsored a ball partly to disprove that "Drinking and Dancing are inseparably connected." Both William Charles M'Kinnon and his *Herald* partner, James Smith, were lecturers at the

of entertaining. In short, Sydney could be a very pleasant assignment for any military officer, noted Lieutenant B.W.A. Sleigh in his journal in 1846. A place of "pretty scenery" with a fine harbour, it afforded the boatman the opportunity for "the healthful exercise of rowing" and gave him ample time to visit the "very pleasant families" he met there:

> There were a few very pleasant families in the town, and at the hospitable house of the Collector of Customs, a most kind-hearted gentlemanly man, with an amiable and ladylike partner, I spent many pleasant hours. The town Major, Sutherland, an accomplished officer deeply read, and an exquisite artist in oil-painting and water-colours and whose productions would reflect credit on our London Exhibitions, was a great acquisition to our little circle. His house, delightfully situated on the opposite side of the river, recently built in the Italian style, was a favourite retreat, where a hearty welcome and a refined tone of conversation were ever to be found, and assured a pleasant evening. Sydney was further fortunate in the residence of one of the most eminent lawyers in the Province, the then Solicitor-General, but who is now promoted to the Bench, where his learning and legal knowledge must prove most valuable: I refer to Judge Dodd. There was also an open house at the Barrack-master's pretty retreat, "Coleby." In this little circle our time was pleasantly diversified, while through the kindness of a Canadian resident, Mr. Bunsinot [Bourinot] I was always provided with the most recent American reprints of the works of favourite English authors.[33]

It would seem that William Charles M'Kinnon — poet, journalist and grandson of the Provincial Secretary — would be a very welcome addition to the pleasant and genteel society described by Sleigh in his 1846 memoirs. However, such was not to be the case. From its first issue, it was clear that *The Cape-Breton Spectator* was to be a Liberal newspaper championing the cause of responsible government and the downfall of the Tory elite in the province. This meant that it attacked the very people whom Sleigh found congenial and cultivated in Sydney, not least of whom was Edmund Dodd whose "learning and legal knowledge" Sleigh so admired. To William Charles M'Kinnon, Dodd represented everything that was wrong with the Tory party, and in a series of editorials in 1847 he attacked the Attorney-General for using a government boat as a pleasure craft for the "aristocracy of Sydney," for blocking democratic freedoms, for resisting Joe Howe's move

---

Temperance Halls. For a description of one of James Smith's texts, see *The Cape-Breton News*, 10 November 1852.

33   "Lieut. (afterwards Lieutenant-Colonel) B.W.A. Sleigh's Description of Sydney, 1846," in C. Bruce Fergusson, ed., *Uniacke's Sketches of Cape Breton* (Halifax, 1958), p. 156-57.

toward responsible government, and for urging in 1839 that the Irish of Low Point be sent off to the "swamps" of the Aroostook to quell disturbances on the North Eastern boundary.[34] In M'Kinnon's editorials, the Conservatives were creatures "belching forth"[35] venom at any head of government who manifested "the slightest disposition to accord justice to the Liberals," and Attorney-General Dodd was one of their central actors:

> In 1844 the curtain rises and discloses Dodd in the act of gazing intently upon a pair of scales. In one scale is a tureen of turtle soup, a flagon of champagne, and a lordling's smiles — in the other, honour, duty, principle, and the interests and wishes of the people. Not long he takes to deliberate — jumping into the scale amongst the turtle soup, etc., up flies the other [scale], and the curtain falls amidst the hisses of an indignant people.[36]

Given the passionate intensity of M'Kinnon's editorials, it is not surprising that he quickly came to the attention of the Halifax pundits. Responding to the Liberal sentiments underlying M'Kinnon's writing, papers like *The Morning Post* of Halifax fastened on to the age and immaturity of the *Spectator* editor and twitted him on the radical tone of his journal. Urging "the young and inexperienced gentleman" to "stroll to some barren rock where he can view the icebergs on the Cape Breton coast,"[37] the *Post* portrayed M'Kinnon as a romantic whose wild fantasies might be nurtured by a diet of raw pork and gothic calisthenics. While the comments were designed to undermine M'Kinnon's credibility and make him appear overwrought and sentimental, they had little influence in cooling his passionate stands on responsible government and equality of opportunity. He called upon "the men who have grown fat and wealthy on the spoils of office" to "put an end to public plunder,"[38] and when the issue seemed to apply to Britain as well as to Nova Scotia, he extended the range of his attack. Listing the tax income received by 339 peers in England, he argued that 83,997 families in Britain could receive £50 per year from those taxes were it not for the perpetuation of privilege in Church and State.[39] He noted that Prince Albert was not content with a mere £30,000 allowance but was trying to accumulate titles and offices

---

34 "Edmund M. Dodd," *The Cape-Breton Spectator*, 22 May 1847.

35 "Conservative Loyalty in British North America," *The Cape Breton Spectator*, 3 April 1847.

36 Editorial, *The Cape-Breton Spectator*, 2 May 1847.

37 "The Cape-Breton Spectator," *The Morning Post*, 5 January 1847. A second taunting editorial appeared in *The Morning Post*, 13 February 1847.

38 Editorial, *The Cape-Breton Spectator*, 22 May 1847.

39 "What the People of England have to Bear — Nice Pickings by Peers and Prelates," *ibid.*, 6 May 1848.

to swell his fortune,[40] and he quoted Halifax correspondent Robin Goodfellow to the effect that the press "is the pride of the freeman and the terror of the despot."[41]

That M'Kinnon saw the *Spectator* as honour-bound to uphold Goodfellow's philosophy is illustrated by his response to a Mechanics' Institute attack on the integrity of the paper in February 1848. Piqued by one of M'Kinnon's reviews, the Mechanics' Institute of Sydney had accused the editor of making "invidious and uncalled for remarks"[42] about one of its lectures. M'Kinnon saw this charge as a flagrant challenge to the freedom of the press. Accusing the "gentlemen" of the Mechanics' Institute of behaving like a "club" and deliberately excluding him from its meetings, he went on to proclaim it the prerogative of the journalist to praise the meritorious and condemn the inadequate. While such a stand reinforced M'Kinnon's Prospectus statement that *The Spectator* would never bend "with mean subserviency to men in authority,"[43] it did nothing to endear the young editor to the power elite of Sydney. Years later it was suggested that M'Kinnon's "strong republican sentiments" and "disloyal" behaviour had so offended Cape Breton society that his newspaper career had suffered accordingly.[44] However true this might have been, it was clear by the summer of 1848 that *The Spectator* was in financial difficulties and that M'Kinnon had lost heavily by investing in it.

If the Tories' dislike of M'Kinnon's newspaper affected its circulation and support, it was nonetheless true that the paper suffered its greatest difficulties because of the poor economic climate in Cape Breton in the famine years of the late 1840s. With crops failing and many families close to starvation, it is not surprising that people had difficulty paying for advertising and for newspapers. However sympathetic M'Kinnon was to the situation of the Islanders,[45] he was forced to request payment from the public in May 1848, to cover his stationer's bill and to pay for the costly new type he had just acquired. With debts of £429 still owing him,[46] he began advertising the sale of his press, type, composing sticks, and office equipment on 3 June 1848,

---

40   "Prince Albert," *ibid.*, 6 May 1848.

41   Editorial note, *ibid.*, 22 January 1848.

42   "The Mechanics' Institute," *ibid.*, 5 February 1848.

43   "Prospectus," *ibid.*, 17 June 1846.

44   Heustis, "Memorials," p. 5.

45   William Charles M'Kinnon was deeply concerned about the growing dependence of Cape Breton on "stock-jobbing" and "contracting." Like Thomas McCulloch in Pictou some 25 years before him, he urged people to turn to the land and be self-sufficient. He ran an agricultural column in *The Cape-Breton Spectator* and called upon Cape Bretoners to turn to farming so they could make their own flour. For representative editorials, see *The Cape-Breton Spectator*, 17 June 1846 and 13 May 1848.

46   "It Must Be Done," *ibid.*, 6 May 1848.

and at the same time threatened to go to law if people did not pay their bills. His passionate editorials had made him controversial in the community before this, but he must have been doubly so when he printed the names of teachers, farmers, and tailors in his paper and included beside their names the amount of money each owed him.[47] Yet in spite of having to resort to this dramatic measure and threaten legal action, M'Kinnon seems to have been able to survive in the newspaper business, and in 1849 he began a new venture under the name, *The Times, and Cape-Breton Spectator.* Differing very little in tone or content from his first journalistic endeavour, this paper also ran into difficulties in the financial environment of the late 1840s. Moreover, many of M'Kinnon's original debtors seem to have carried over into this venture and to have added to his liabilities. Finally to make a new start, M'Kinnon decided to dissolve the *Times,* adopt James Smith as a partner,[48] and begin *The Commercial Herald* of Sydney.

Edmund Dodd had once declared in a political gathering that he would crush *The Cape-Breton Spectator,*[49] but he needed to take no such action against *The Commercial Herald* when it began publication. From the beginning, the paper seemed less controversial and more culturally-oriented than M'Kinnon's previous ventures. The editor's association with a partner and his increasing involvement with the temperance movement may have had something to do with this new moderation, but it is more likely that M'Kinnon had begun to regard his newspaper work in a different light as he began to think of writing as a professional career. He had always published poems and sketches from British and American journals in his newspapers, but he now saw *The Commercial Herald* as a potential vehicle for regional literature and for his own creative writing. His novel *Castine, A Legend of Cape Breton* began to appear in the paper as a serial in January of 1850,[50] and

---

47   *Ibid.,* 15 July 1848.

48   James Smith was a fellow Methodist and, like M'Kinnon, was active in the temperance movement. After leaving the *Herald,* he taught reading, writing, arithmetic, grammar, algebra, and Latin to 130 pupils in Sydney Mines (see "Schools, Cape Breton 1852," RG 14, Cape Breton County, PANS). Smith had twelve books in his library in 1852. There are indications in *The Commercial Herald* that M'Kinnon was the editor and probably the driving force behind the paper.

49   "Township of Sydney," repr. from *The Eastern Chronicle* in *The Cape-Breton Spectator,* 22 May 1847.

50   *Castine, A Legend of Cape Breton* was serialized in *The Commercial Herald* in January and February 1850. It was reprinted in *The Eastern Chronicle* of Pictou ("by permission") from 18 April until 23 May 1850, and was accompanied by an editorial note on 18 April 1850. The novel was subsequently serialized in *The Waverley Magazine* of Boston ("written for *The Waverley Magazine*") as *St. Castine. A Legend of Cape Breton* (the title used in the book version). It appeared in *The Waverley Magazine* on 19 October 1850. Between 17 and 21 September 1880, *The Morning Herald* of Halifax began to reprint *St. Castine. A Legend of Cape Breton* but did not complete the serialization.

although it was published anonymously, it was undoubtedly clear to most readers that M'Kinnon was the author. An editorial note encouraged people to save copies of the newspaper so they would have a complete run of the story and could read it to "advantage," and on 26 January 1850, M'Kinnon made an announcement that the *Herald* office would publish the romance in book form once enough subscribers had committed themselves to the project. Agents in Halifax, St. John's (Newfoundland), Sydney and rural Cape Breton were designated to collect subscriptions for this "most thrilling and popular romance ever written in Nova Scotia."[51] At some point between March and September 1850, *St. Castine* appeared in book form as a Sydney imprint.[52]

Shrewdly following a proven formula for his first venture into fiction, M'Kinnon organized *St. Castine* around Sir Walter Scott's practice of showing two societies in conflict, one ascendant and one descendant. Like Scott's work, *St. Castine* also had clearly defined opposing forces, an interesting villain, a heroine waiting to be rescued, and vivid, muscular action. However, unlike many of his contemporaries who had reworked Scott's conventions into yet another version of medieval or Tudor history, William Charles M'Kinnon turned to the relatively recent past of his own island of Cape Breton for inspiration. *St. Castine* is set in Louisbourg "about a hundred years ago"[53] when Wolfe, Amherst, and Boscowan are moored off the coast preparing for an attack on the fortress. The central figure in this historical adventure is Henry Runnington Beauclerc, a British spy who has penetrated the governor's palace at Louisbourg disguised as Castine, chief of the Micmac. His dangerous mission and the effectiveness of his disguise bring an element of exoticism to M'Kinnon's action:

> With a savage exclamation of pain he [the Lieutenant] looked up and beside him saw, a man, whose olive complexion and black plume bespoke him a Micmac chieftan. His proportions were gigantic, his height being about six feet three inches and his breadth of chest and shoulders corresponding. His raven hair fell thick over a high forehead and a curved nose, black brows, and eyes that gleamed with each changing shade of light, gave a Gladiator like expression to his features. He wore a scarlet jacket, braided with horsehair, a blue cloth cap and plume, and was armed merely with a scalping knife.[54]

---

51   Notice, *The Commercial Herald*, 12 January 1850; "Will Be Published," *ibid.*, 23 March 1850.

52   The advertisement for subscribers was still being published in *The Commercial Herald* as late as 23 March 1850. Sometime between that date and M'Kinnon's departure for Boston in September, *St. Castine* appeared in book form in Sydney.

53   William Charles M'Kinnon, *St. Castine; A Legend of Cape Breton* (Sydney, 1850), p. 3.

54   *Ibid.*, pp. 7-8.

It is clear that certain conventions of popular romance are being developed in this episode as M'Kinnon introduces his hero to his audience. The "high brow" suggests the intelligence of Beauclerc, the "curved nose" and "gleaming black eyes" indicate his intensity, and his height and size conjure up possibilities of heroic feats of strength. The over-all blackness of Beauclerc's hair, brow, and expression suggests the melancholy of Byron's passionate heroes, and the reference to his being armed "merely with a scalping knife" illustrates both his ferocity and his warrior-like courage. All M'Kinnon's characters in *St. Castine* are given a distinctive identity through such physical or external descriptions. Women are fair, passive, and prone to fainting at the slightest sign of danger. Men are manly if they are heroes and lecherous if they are villains. Obviously, then, readers did not expect a novel of interiority when they bought William Charles M'Kinnon's work, but instead wanted the high adventure, blood and thunder, tender romance, and black and white moralism that *St. Castine* represents. The only deviation from this pattern occurs when the author tries to intrude a philosophical observation or a social comment into the action, but ever conscious of his audience, he apologetically retreats from his story behind the plumes and exploits of his heroes: "But there is no use in moralizing. In reading a work of this kind, I generally skip over all the moralizing and get on with the narrative parts. I suppose my readers do the same; consequently there is no use in writing what will never be read."[55]

Because it adheres to simple conventions, a novel like *St. Castine* remains a fast-paced, multi-coloured panorama of intrigue, mistaken identity, treachery by night, and hand-to-hand combat. The action culminates in the fall of Louisbourg and Wolfe's order that the city be dismantled ("I have sworn that the plough and the harrow shall go over Louisbourg, and as I have sworn, so shall it be!").[56] The noble hero Beauclerc survives and wins his lady; the villains are killed fairly in battle; and fraternal bonds are cemented as Beauclerc swears fidelity to his half-brother, the real Castine. To emphasize the new order, Wolfe is given the closing words in this fictional drama, symbolizing by his very presence the restoration of harmony and the triumph of British hegemony.

St. Castine heralded the beginning of a series of similar fictions by William Charles M'Kinnon. Incorporating quotations from Byron, Scott, N.P. Willis, Bulwer-Lytton, and Captain Marryat into their narratives, stories like *Francis, or Pirate Cove: A Legend of Cape Breton*,[57] *Child of the Sun*,[58] and

55   *Ibid.*, p. 50.

56   *Ibid.*, p. 71.

57   W.C. M'Kinnon, *Francis, or Pirate Cove. A Legend of Cape Breton* (Halifax, 1851).

58   W.C. M'Kinnon, "The Child of the Sun: A Legend of Peru," *The Waverley Magazine*, II (5 October 1850), pp. 33-34.

The Rival Brothers of the Revolution[59] all rely on the conventions of popular romance while adhering to the Scott pattern of showing two powers in conflict at a critical moment in their history. The challenges experienced by M'Kinnon's fictional characters unfold in the shadow of these great events, demanding the heightened courage and strong moral commitment expected of romantic heroes. M'Kinnon's use of documentary evidence and his introduction of historical figures like General Wolfe, Benedict Arnold and Francis Pisarro offset the costume-drama elements of his fiction. His primary concern was always to entertain, however, and historical accuracy is therefore sublimated to that purpose. Nonetheless, where he could, M'Kinnon used fact as the basis of his story and developed a series of romantic embellishments around that core.

One of the best illustrations of M'Kinnon's technique in employing history as the basis of a tale is *The Midnight Murder. A Legend of Cape Breton* published in *The Commercial Herald* on 23 March 1850. Based on the Flahaven murder case in Sydney in 1833, the story is embellished by the addition of colourful dialect characters (a Yankee sailor and an intoxicated Gaelic backlander), a tangled tale of thwarted love, and several dramatic subplots. The actual murder occurred in Sydney when Charlotte Flahaven and two sailor cohorts murdered her husband, John Flahaven, a tavern keeper. He had just brought an ox from Little Bras d'Or to Sydney when the men untied the beast and sent its owner in hot pursuit. While Flahaven looked for the animal, the sailors waylaid the man and killed him.[60] The suspicions of Flahavens' sixteen-year old daughter eventually led to the murderers' being arrested by Magistrate John M'Kinnon, father of the author William Charles M'Kinnon. "Fettered by the plain facts," notes the writer, he therefore cannot assume the fictional pose and the detachment usually afforded a novelist. Instead, the "writer of these pages" has been "in converse with the magistrate spoken of," and faced with the facts from this "old half-pay officer of a disbanded regiment," can do little to change the story in a scene so "local" and with events so "recent."[61]

In spite of M'Kinnon's claim that *The Midnight Murder* is more fact than fiction, the story gives every impression of being a lurid gothic tale employing disguise, entombment, blood-lust, and lechery as devices to frighten and titillate the reader. That M'Kinnon is consciously playing on the audience's expectation of such a tale is obvious in his reference at the beginning of the story to "horrible events" and to *The Mysteries of Paris.*

59   W.C. M'Kinnon, "The Rival Brothers of the Revolution. A Tale," *The Waverley Magazine*, II (26 October 1850), pp. 57-58; repr. in *The Eastern Chronicle*, 5-19 December 1850.

60   MacKinnon, *Old Sydney*, pp. 59-60.

61   W.C. M'Kinnon, *The Midnight Murder. A Legend of Cape Breton*, *The Waverley Magazine*, II (16 November 1850), pp. 83, 88.

Having successfully established the image of Eugene Sue as a mock ideal, M'Kinnon proceeds to weave effective descriptions of North Sydney and pungent asides about society into the narrative in order to distract the reader from the imminent rapes and dismembered bodies that punctuate the action. His honest Gaelic backlander ("for in those days, a Backlander sometimes did receive money for his shingles and puncheons"), his narrator's down-to-earth character ("Our feelings are natural, the path of duty artificial, and what society in one age tells you is your duty, the next age annuls") and the villains' colourful language ("solemncholy," "absquatulate," "dunghill churl," and "moccasin preaching") all function as grounding devices to offset the melodrama and structural disorganization of the author's tale. M'Kinnon's handling of time occasionally creates confusion, and his central characters are always one dimensional.[62] Nonetheless, the narrator's energy in telling the tale and his reluctance to take the atrocities too seriously go far in explaining the popularity of the novel in Boston and Sydney in 1850.[63]

St. Castine and *The Midnight Murder* were originally written to boost the sales and popularity of the Sydney *Herald,* but in April and May 1850, *The Eastern Chronicle* of Pictou also serialized *St. Castine* on the mainland. This attention to M'Kinnon's fiction came at an opportune time, for in May 1850 James Smith announced that he was withdrawing from *The Commercial Herald* and from his partnership with William Charles M'Kinnon. Noting that the *Herald* was no longer an economically viable proposition, Smith argued that public goodwill was not "sufficient to remunerate the publishers for their labour and outlay."[64] Only two Sydney merchants were paying for advertising in the paper, and job work and subscriptions were not adequate to absorb the costs of maintenance. Smith and M'Kinnon were spending approximately £250 per annum on the journal and were realizing only £70-100 in return. Lamenting that Cape Bretoners regarded a newspaper as a superfluity rather than a necessity, Smith revealed that he now found the publication of the *Herald* too "soul-wearying and profitless" to pursue. Although planning to travel "the shore of some distant land" at the time of the announcement, Smith eventually became a schoolmaster in Sydney Mines and an active participant in the temperance movement in the Sydneys.

Although the Smith-M'Kinnon partnership was dissolved on 25 May 1850, Smith seemed to think that William Charles M'Kinnon would carry on with the editing and publishing of the newspaper. However, no copies of the paper have survived after that date, and it is possible that M'Kinnon decided to

---

62 *The Midnight Murder*, pp. 81, 82, 83.

63 *The Midnight Murder* was reputed to have had a readership of 13,000 people in "Boston alone, last summer," *The Cape-Breton News*, 24 May 1851 [rpt. from *The Eastern Chronicle* of Pictou]. It first appeared in *The Commercial Herald* of Sydney, 23 March 1850.

64 "To the Readers of The *Herald,*" *The Commercial Herald*, 25 May 1850.

pursue a new career once the partnership with Smith was dissolved. That this career was to be a literary one is clear from M'Kinnon's actions in the next few months. Demanding that all *Spectator* and *Herald* notes be paid by the first of September and disposing of his house in Sydney,[65] M'Kinnon embarked for Boston to try his fortune in the publishing world there. By October 1850 he had managed to become a contributor to the increasingly popular *Waverley Magazine*,[66] a journal admirably suited to someone of his historical sensibility. Between October and November, M'Kinnon contributed *The Child of the Sun: A Legend of Peru, St. Castine: A Legend of Cape Breton, The Rival Brothers of the Revolution, The Midnight Murder,* and a poem entitled "Kissing" to the *Waverley Magazine*.[67] Two of the novels had appeared earlier in Cape Breton, but the *Waverley* presented them as if they had been written exclusively for the magazine. In all likelihood, this subterfuge represents William Charles M'Kinnon's own shrewd assessment of the competitiveness of the American literary market, and it is obvious from *The Rival Brothers of the Revolution* that he quickly recognized the kind of story that would have a mass market appeal in the United States. A pro-Whig tale set in the United States during the War of Independence, *The Rival Brothers* paints the Loyalists and the British as effete, aristocratic and cruel. Subsequently circulated in Nova Scotia in *The Eastern Chronicle* of Pictou,[68] the story seems a contradictory one to have been written by the grandson of a Loyalist and the son of a British officer. However, it was the kind of narrative that would have a direct appeal to patriotic Americans and for that reason would be eminently saleable to *The Waverley Magazine.*

What direction M'Kinnon's fiction might have taken had he remained in the United States is in the realm of conjecture, but he was no doubt encouraged in his American literary ambitions by *The Waverley Magazine's* claim that he was "a gentleman of rare talents" who "bids fair to become one of the best novelists of the day."[69] However, shortly after *The Cape-Breton News* had reprinted this encomium in Sydney for the benefit of M'Kinnon's former readers, ill health forced the young author to return to Nova Scotia and a less advantageous literary environment than the one he had encountered in Boston. As had earlier been the case in Sydney, M'Kinnon turned to

---

65 "Must Be Paid," and "Grammar School," *The Cape-Breton News,* 31 August 1850.

66 *The Waverley Magazine* was established by Moses A. Dow in Boston in 1850 and continued into the twentieth century. It was devoted to "Tales, Poetry, Music, The Drama, and Useful Information."

67 W.C. M'Kinnon, "Kissing," *The Waverley Magazine,* II (2 November 1850), p. 72.

68 W.C. M'Kinnon, "The Rival Brothers of the Revolution, From *The Waverley Magazine.* A Tale," *Eastern Chronicle,* 5-19 December 1850.

69 *The Cape Breton News,* 14 December 1850. My thanks to Beryl Davis for drawing my attention to this issue of the paper in the Beaton Archives in Sydney.

newspaper editing as a way of supporting himself in Nova Scotia. Throughout 1851 he seems to have conducted the Halifax *New Era* for William Cunnabel, a fellow Methodist whose family had been active in printing and publishing since the 1820s. Appearing tri-weekly under the masthead "Westward the Star of Empire Makes Its Way," the *New Era* promised to represent the "views and feelings of the British North American Colonist,"[70] a sentiment consistent with M'Kinnon's nationalist and populist stand in his Cape Breton newspapers. While the *New Era* claimed to be independent in politics, the Liberal affiliation of its editor was not only well known in Halifax but also was given definition when in April 1851 M'Kinnon offered himself for nomination as a Liberal candidate in Victoria County in Cape Breton. In an open address "To the Electors of the County of Victoria" in June 1851, M'Kinnon announced to potential electors that by "strict attention, energy and vigilance," he would "advance your interests and successfully advocate your claims." While he was clearly at a disadvantage in mounting his campaign from the distance of Halifax, he felt hopeful that the electors' knowledge of him "from an early age" would stand him in good stead and enable him to "represent some section of my native Island."[71]

The amount of time M'Kinnon could devote to his campaign in Victoria County must have been highly limited, for throughout the spring and summer of 1851 he was not only engaged in journalistic activities in Halifax but also was involved in preparing *St. George, or, the Canadian League* and *Francis, or Pirate Cove* for publication. *The Cape-Breton News* of 29 March 1851 drew the attention of its readers to the impending availability of *St. George,*[72] an "original novel" purporting to "contain upwards of seventy chapters." To be sold for a dollar per copy, it was to be distributed in Saint John, Halifax, Sydney, North Sydney, Arichat, and St. John's. That M'Kinnon was still writing the novel during the month of April is clear from a similar advertisement appearing in *The Cape-Breton News* on 26 April, for in that announcement the work had grown from 70 chapters to 110. By May 1851, the novel was being advertised in Pictou with full support from *The Eastern Chronicle*, the newspaper which had serialized *Castine* and *The Rival Brothers of the Revolution*. Remembering *Castine* as a novel evidencing "much skill and power of graphic delineation on the part of the writer,"[73] *The Eastern Chronicle* went on to describe the success of M'Kinnon's *Midnight*

70 Gertrude E.N. Tratt, *A Survey and Listing of Nova Scotia Newspapers: 1752-1957* (Halifax, 1979). I have not been able to locate any copies of this newspaper to examine M'Kinnon's contribution to it.

71 "To The Electors of the County of Victoria," *The Cape-Breton News*, 28 June 1851.

72 *Ibid.*, 29 March 1851.

73 "Encourage Native Talent," *ibid.*, 24 May 1851.

Murder in Boston and to encourage its readers to support "native talent" by buying *St. George*.

William Charles M'Kinnon no doubt felt that *St. George* would be completed in June well before the Victoria County nominating meeting, for on 16 June 1851, *The Novascotian* was advertising the novel as "in press" at five shillings per copy.[74] The newspaper urged "parties wishing to subscribe" to the work to express interest immediately, for the "first edition" of this "new and thrilling historical novel" was being published in a limited edition. The small run of the book suggests M'Kinnon's lack of success in attracting subscribers, and there seems to be little support for the announcement in July that *St. George* was also being published in the United States.[75] After months of newspaper advertisements had appeared promising the imminent release of the novel, *St. George* finally was published with Fuller of Halifax in early 1852, a good eight or nine months after the announced date of publication. Whether the delay was caused by financial problems or by indecisiveness remains unclear, but it may well have been the chequered publication history of *St. George* that influenced M'Kinnon to withdraw from the political arena in August 1851. Appearing before the constituents of Victoria County at Baddeck, he "addressed the electors" but "declined being put in nomination, or soliciting their suffrages."[76] Instead, he seems to have again focused on writing and editing as an outlet for his energies and awaited the publication of *St. George* to give his literary career the impetus it needed for publicity and success.

In spite of the difficulties caused by the delay in publishing *St. George*, the advertisements at least had the advantage of keeping M'Kinnon's name before the literary public throughout 1851. Moreover, he received some attention as a novelist when *Francis, or Pirate Cove* appeared in the *British North American* in July and was published in book form later in that year.[77] A rather melodramatic story about the activities of Jordan the Pirate off the coast of New England and Cape Breton, *Francis, or Pirate Cove* was vintage M'Kinnon in the way it developed a tale of romance and derring-do against a convincingly-sketched historical background. However, it was in many respects a less successful effort than M'Kinnon's four-part narrative poem "Ballad," published in the *Mayflower* in August 1851. Following the author's usual approach to historical narrative by purporting to be "based on fact,"

---

74 *The Novascotian*, 16 July 1851.

75 *The Cape-Breton News*, 12 July 1851.

76 "Victoria County," *ibid.*, 30 August 1851.

77 I have not been able to locate the issues of *The British North American* containing *Francis, or Pirate Cove*. However, an item in *The Cape-Breton News*, 12 July 1851, indicates that the story was then running in *The British North American*. It was later published by *The British North American* office as a book.

"Ballad" counterpointed the domesticity of rural life in Hungary with the havoc of war during the Kossuth drive for self-determination. The theme of justice so commonly explored in Sir Walter Scott's work found expression here as well, and the poem concluded by taking Madeleine and her Kossuth lover away from the tyranny of their homeland to the freedom of America. However, in spite of this very North American ending, the emphasis of the poem lay on courage, idealism, and the carnage of war. With muscular, action-stressed verbs and strong rhymes, M'Kinnon caught the chaotic rhythm and confusion of battle:

> And the wounded horses reeling go
>   Through trampled fields of corn —
>   And friend and foe
>   Rush to and fro,
>   Trampling the forms of the dead below —
>   And the victor, flushed with triumph's glow,
>   Exults in his work of death and woe —
>   And mercy laughs to scorn![78]

In spite of the literary congeniality of Halifax, M'Kinnon returned to Cape Breton in 1852 to continue writing at home and to look for a satisfying career. His hopes for literary success were undoubtedly reliant on the favourable reception of *St. George, or, The Canadian League.* However, it was clear by April 1852 that the public found the tale confusing and overly long. In his preface to the two-volume work, M'Kinnon had tried to document his claim that a secret revolutionary league had existed in Lower Canada at the time of the 1837 rebellion, and following the pattern of his other novels, he had used a germ of historical fact to focus and unify the book. As a result Louis Joseph Papineau and William Lyon Mackenzie appear in the secret meetings and intrigues which make up M'Kinnon's complicated plot, but they are far less interesting as characters than is the author's revengeful villain, Rodolphe. Assuming a number of disguises destined to confuse all but the most careful reader, Rodolphe tries to control his peers through hypnotism (called "biology" or "magnetism" in the novel). By the conclusion of the book he has wreaked havoc on a series of lives and is himself a candidate for the hand of nemesis. Not surprisingly, perhaps, these melodramatic sequences seemed overwrought to a local historian like Mary Jane Katzmann of *The Provincial,* and in a review of *St. George* she dismissed "its windings and contradictions" as subjects for only the most "peculiar mind."[79]

---

78 "Ballad," *The Mayflower,* I (August 1851), pp. 101-06.

79 *St. George; or, The Canadian League. A Tale of the Outbreak,* in *The Provincial* (April 1852), pp. 146-48. For a modern discussion of M'Kinnon's *St. George,* see Carole Gerson,

In spite of the set-back to his literary career that the poor response to *St. George* represented, M'Kinnon continued to write throughout 1852 and 1853. Most significant, perhaps, were his contributions to *The Wesleyan*, the religious newspaper that increasingly became a literary outlet for him as he strengthened his commitment to the Methodist Church. The poems published in the journal between November 1852 and August 1853 were personal and domestic in tone, often expressing admiration for public figures like Silas Tertius Rand or for private family members like M'Kinnon's brother or sister. At the same time, M'Kinnon actively participated in the lecturing life of Sydney, giving a talk to the Mechanics' Institute on January 12th on "the Prosperity of the Age" and another on January 19th on "Phonography or Phonetic Short Hand."[80] A plan to teach phonograpy in Sydney does not seem to have materialized, perhaps because M'Kinnon's spiritual experience at a Methodist watchnight service in Sydney in January had already convinced him that his future lay with the Methodist ministry. From February 2nd onward, most temperance meetings described in *The Cape-Breton News* make some mention of M'Kinnon's having addressed the society, and there is every suggestion in these same accounts that the Sydneys were at this time undergoing a vigorous period of Wesleyan revivalism. One correspondent attending a Methodist service in March 1853 objected to cheering and footstamping after the singing and the musical presentations and felt that topboots were unsuitable for social occasions.[81] However, such cavilling does not seem to have daunted the spirit of enthusiasm felt in Sydney Wesleyan circles as people responded to the preaching of the Reverend Robert Crane, a Methodist cleric who had arrived in Sydney in July 1852.[82] Significantly, when Crane left Cape Breton in the "Susanna" in May 1853 to attend the Methodist District Meeting in Charlottetown, he was accompanied by William Charles M'Kinnon as a probationary minister.[83]

Once embarked on a clerical course, William Charles M'Kinnon looked back on his fiction-writing career as a frivolous and embarrassing segment of his life. In a fit of remorse he tried to destroy every copy of his novels that he

---

"Shaping the English-Canadian Novel," Ph.D. thesis, University of British Columbia, 1977, pp. 189-90.

80   *The Cape Breton News* advertised M'Kinnon's lecture on "The Prosperity of The Age" on 12 January 1853. The same newspaper described his address on "Phonography or Phonetic Shorthand" on 19 January 1853. This brief article indicated that M'Kinnon would be willing to teach phonography were there enough interest in Sydney.

81   "Temperance Soirée," *The Cape-Breton News*, 2 March 1853.

82   *Ibid.*, 5 July 1851.

83   Under "Passengers" in *ibid.*, 18 May 1853, there appears this notice: "In the Susanna for Halifax, Rev. Mr. Crane, lady, and infant; Mr. W.C. M'Kinnon." Another note in the same issue indicates that the Reverend Mr. Crane's destination is the District Meeting of the Wesleyan Methodist Church in Charlottetown.

could find during the next nine years, throwing himself into his career as a minister with all the passion and intensity that had once enlivened his political editorials and his fictional romances. Congregations in Bedeque, Canso, Guysborough, and Middle Musquodoboit spoke of his eloquence in the pulpit and his tireless dedication to the service of the church. The scholarly attitudes that had once taken him into studies of literature, history, ornithology, and astronomy now found expression in theological arguments and in the publication of sermons such as *The Papacy: The Sacrifice of the Mass* (1859), and *The Divine Sovereignty* (1861).[84] Although traces of the literary William Charles M'Kinnon emerged briefly in these sermons in references to Byron and Shakespeare, there is little indication after 1853 that he wrote anything other than expository prose. A series of pulpit sketches, a study of Musquodobit Valley fossils and geology, an essay on Sir William Dawson and three chapters of a study of Nova Scotia geology all appeared in *The Wesleyan Magazine* between 1860 and 1862,[85] so that in every sense M'Kinnon seems to have channelled his love of romance into a dedication to his new vocation. Writing to Joseph Howe in 1856, M'Kinnon noted that Howe's devotion to his country and his poetical temperament had inspired him in his youth and had supported him in his editorial battles for responsible government. Now a clergyman in Bedeque, Prince Edward Island, he found it his duty to fight another kind of battle and to repay Howe for his previous inspiration and encouragement by offering him the solace of prayer and spiritual advice.[86]

M'Kinnon was ordained in 1857[87] and shortly afterward married Miriam Matilda Crane of Pugwash, the daughter of a deceased Wesleyan minister.

---

84 Rev. W.C. M'Kinnon, *The Papacy: The Sacrifice of the Mass* (Halifax, 1859); and *The Divine Sovereignty. A Sermon on Jeremiah XVIII, 6* (Halifax, 1861).

85 The "Chapters on Geology" that appear in *The Provincial Wesleyan* on 5, 12, and 26 February 1862 are not signed by M'Kinnon but it is almost a certainty that they are his work. M'Kinnon had been working on a study of Nova Scotian geology (Chapter 1 mentions Sydney) before his death, and according to G.O. Heustis in his memorial to M'Kinnon, some of his work on geology was published just before his death (on 22 March 1862). There were very few others of his expertise in geology who would publish on the subject in *The Provincial Wesleyan*, a Methodist religious paper. In the last years of his life, M'Kinnon directed nearly all of his writing to this journal.

86 W.C. M'Kinnon to Joseph Howe, December 1856, Joseph Howe Papers, PANS Microfilm, vol. 2, pp. 801-10. A second letter written on 11 April 1857 appears on pp. 879-84. I am grateful to Beryl Davies of Glace Bay for drawing my attention to M'Kinnon's correspondence with Howe.

87 M'Kinnon was examined for the ministry in 1856 but for undisclosed reasons was continued on trial. See "A Journal of the Proceedings of the Nova Scotia East or Charlottetown District held at Guysborough commencing on Thursday, 22 May 1856, at nine o'clock a.m." in the Archives, Pine Hill Divinity Hall, Halifax. M'Kinnon was received into the ministry the following year.

They served the Methodist congregation at Middle Musquodobit for three years before tuberculosis began to erode William Charles M'Kinnon's health. M'Kinnon and his family moved to Shelburne in the summer of 1861 to take up a new charge, but he was too ill to fulfil his circuit responsibilities after November of that year. He died on 22 March 1862, leaving his wife and two infant children.[88] His wife died the following November, lamented in a poem in *The Wesleyan* as a woman of "gentle Christian graces."[89] Their two children, William and John, were supported by the children's fund of the Methodist Church until 1874,[90] and John is shown as living in Pugwash with his maternal grandmother in the 1871 census.[91]

After William Charles M'Kinnon's death, testimonials were sent to *The Wesleyan* from all over the province. Brother Leonard Gaetz, who had replaced him in Middle Musquodobit, spoke of M'Kinnon's "noble heaven-inspired actions" being indelibly stamped "upon the brilliant drama of colonial Methodism."[92] G.O. Heustis wrote a long biographical sketch of his life and affectionately described him as a scholar so engrossed in his theological readings that he once walked a mile with his horse from Canso to Guysborough before realizing that the animal had slipped out of its halter and was grazing somewhere behind.[93] And the Reverend Joseph Angwin, looking back on the history of Methodism in Cape Breton, recalled the eloquent young probationer who had preached so effectively to his countrymen in Gaelic.[94]

In the final assessment of William Charles M'Kinnon's place in Nova Scotia history, however, it is as a cultural figure, not as a cleric, that he has lasting importance. At a time when the literature of other nations was flooding Nova Scotia, he recognized that his province and country had a history as storied and as proud as that of any. This does not mean that he failed to see Nova Scotia's place in a wider historical spectrum, nor does it mean that he ignored the continuing links between the old world and the new.

88   See "Shelburne Circuit," *The Provincial Wesleyan*, 19 March 1862; "Obituary Notices," *ibid.*, 16 April 1862; "Obituary Notices. Memorials of the late Rev. Mr. W.C. M'Kinnon, *ibid.*, 18 June 1862; "Cemeteries: Shelburne: 1785-1912," Microfilm: Cemeteries, F7, PANS.

89   "Lines on the Death of Mrs. W.C. M'Kinnon," *The Provincial Wesleyan*, 24 December 1862.

90   "Children's Fund — 1862-1863 of the Conference of Eastern British America: 1856-1874," Truro District, Pine Hill Divinity Hall.

91   James F. Smith, *The History of Pugwash* (Oxford, 1978), p. 157.

92   Leonard Gaetz, "Middle Musquodobit Circuit," *The Provincial Wesleyan*, 14 May 1862.

93   Heustis, *The Provincial Wesleyan*, 18 June 1862.

94   Joseph Angwin, *Methodism in Cape Breton, 1789-1914. A Retrospect* (Sydney Mines, 1914), pp. 45-46. There is some evidence that William Charles M'Kinnon also wrote poetry in Gaelic.

Reporting on a meeting of the Highland Society in Baddeck in 1847, he had noted that the group was gathering in a community "where those who cherish fond recollections of their father land — the land of 'Brown heath and shaggy wood' — that Land made classic by the song of Robert Burns — and immortal by the halo of Romance thrown over it by the strains of Walter Scott — had an opportunity of expressing the warm feelings that exist this side the Atlantic. The affair, we understood, came off well — but we regret not being present — for we, too, confess with pride that we have deep sympathies in common with Scotchmen and Scotland."[95]

However, in spite of being able to identify with Scotland and his own traditions, William Charles M'Kinnon always felt first and foremost a Cape Bretoner and a Nova Scotian. Thus, he wanted to do for his homeland what Sir Walter Scott and Edward Bulwer-Lytton had done for theirs by imaginatively interpreting the country's history in entertaining fictions that developed a sense of place and a pride in the past. "America has been scoffed at because her history abounds not with old-time events as do the records of the Eastern World," he noted in *The Child of the Sun*. "They say we cannot turn to such fields for contemplation as those afforded by old Cheops pyramids — by the rocks of Thermopylae — the grass-grown mounds of Troy.... But...who will deny, that when years have rolled away and the immediate memory of their occurrence shall have died in men's bosoms...that the history of the last century shall not afford as proud material for the writer's pen and the poet's song, as Europe can produce."[96] In writing this, William Charles M'Kinnon was encouraging North Americans to recognize that their country had imaginatively come of age. Although he may have admired and followed Sir Walter Scott, he meant Cape Breton and Nova Scotia when he wrote his historical poems and stories under the headnote: "This is my own, my native land."

---

95 "Doings at Baddeck," *The Cape-Breton Spectator*, 13 May 1847.

96 W.C. M'Kinnon, "The Child of the Sun: A Legend of Peru," *The Waverley Magazine*, 5 October 1850.

Sailing for the Goldfields:
The Ballarat-Maritime Provinces Connection

Throughout the spring and summer of 1852, advertisements appeared in the newspapers of the Maritime Provinces announcing imminent sailings for the goldfields of Australia. "For Australia Ho!," "For The Rich Gold Regions of Australia!" and "Australian Gold Mine! For Port Philip and Sydney" were not isolated bannerlines as captains vied for passengers, editors speculated on the adventure of the goldfields, and reporters described the fanfare of wharfside departures.[1] The Australian Company of Saint John was typical of share corporations formed to fund gold-seeking ventures; the "Ariadne" of the same city was built on speculation to ply the Australian trade; the *New Brunswick Reporter* of Fredericton published excerpts from Cunningham's *Two Years In New South Wales* (1837) for public edification; and calls went out to the young men of communities as diverse as Charlottetown, Sydney, Halifax, Saint John, Pictou, Yarmouth and Barrington to join expeditions to Ballarat and environs.[2] Under the bannerline "Australia! Australia!! — Highly Important!!!," W.H. Bashford of Saint John urged "Persons preparing for Australia" to purchase Montgomery Martin's *History of The British Colonies* so they would be adequately informed, and the National Loan Fund Life Assurance Society ran advertisements inviting "Parties proceeding to Australia" to insure themselves with the firm before setting off.[3] In short, in the spring and summer of 1852, the Maritime Provinces of Canada were seized by antipodes fever as the lure of the California gold rush of the 1840s receded and the promise of Ballarat hovered tantalizingly in the air.

The reasons why young Maritimers were tempted to leave their homeland and travel half-way around the world in search of gold were several. Certainly, as with the California gold rush, Australia offered excitement and adventure, a point reiterated by various editors as they observed the exodus of young men from the region. Phrases like "spirit of enterprise," "love of adventure," and "success at their El Dorado" inform their columns as they mourn the loss of "the best blood of the country,"[4] and the *Novascotian* of Halifax struck a typical note of moralism and frustration on 5 July 1852 when it remarked on yet another clipper departing the city for Port Philip:

---

1   *Novascotian* (Halifax), 13 September 1852; *Morning News* (Saint John), 21, 24 May 1852.

2   "For Australia," *Morning News*, 12, 14, 21 April 1852; "Literature. Emigration to New South Wales," *The New Brunswick Reporter* (Fredericton), 25 June 1852.

3   *Morning News*, 28 May, 2 June 1852.

4   "Immigration and Emigration. Nova Scotians go to Australia," *Novascotian*, 5 July 1852; "Departure of the 'Aurora'," *ibid.*, 27 September 1852.

. . . there are young men going out in the *Chebucto*, who, impregnated with the spirit of adventure, have thrown up eligible situations and promising prospects to gratify it, and the hope of improving their fortunes. Heaven grant that all those on the eve of leaving us for the antipodes, may be as successful as the most sanguine temperament can anticipate. What has induced them to leave countries so full of future promise, as these northern provinces undoubtedly are, is of course nobody's business but their own. If they were serfs of the Czar, he would *compel* them to remain at home. But in all free countries this restless love of change of locality is a characteristic feature of society....[5]

While the *Novascotian* was undoubtedly correct in identifying a "restless love of change" as one reason for the outmigration of Maritimers to the Australian goldfields, it was wrong in suggesting that the young had a prosperous future if they remained in the Maritimes. Unquestionably, the most compelling motivation for the exodus from the province was economic. Throughout the 1840s, the fortunes of the Maritime region had fluctuated, but by the late 1840s and early 1850s, international banking constrictions, crop failures in Nova Scotia, uncontrolled Irish immigration after the potato famine of 1846-48, the repeal of the Corn Laws, Britain's reduction of timber preferences for the colonies, and Britain's abolition of the Navigation Acts had all had a dramatic impact on the Maritime economy.[6] This was particularly true in New Brunswick, as W.S. MacNutt has pointed out, for the province relied heavily on preferences for the sale of timber in British markets and on the buoyancy of its timber merchants for the vitality of its shipbuilding industry.[7] Symptomatic of the financial malaise afflicting New Brunswick commercial ventures after the loss of preferences was the fate of the Saint John clipper, the Marco Polo. Launched on 17 April 1851 for the timber trade, she was sold only two voyages later to the Black Ball line of Liverpool to service the lucrative passenger route between England and the Australian goldfields. The pride of the European-Australian run, the "Marco Polo" cut two months off the return trip on her first voyage out and, proudly for her Saint John builders, earned the reputation of being the fastest ship in the world.[8] Such honours were dubious, however, when they represented the loss of talent, money, and ambition from the Atlantic region, and newspapers

5   *Ibid.*, 5 July 1852.

6   W.S. MacNutt, *The Atlantic Provinces* (Toronto, 1965), pp. 234-37.

7   *Ibid.*, p. 235.

8   Esther Clark Wright, *Saint John Ships and their Builders* (Wolfville, N.S., 1976), pp. 80-84; Charles A. Armour and Thomas Lackey, *Sailing Ships of the Maritimes* (Toronto, 1975), pp. 58-59.

like the Saint John *Morning News* and the Fredericton *Reporter* were typical in publishing mournful editorials on this theme. "It is thought by our operatives generally," noted the *Morning News* in the "State of Business," that business in St. John is so bad, and the prospect of better times so remote, that numbers of our young and most active men are making arrangements to leave their homes for Australia, and the United States, in expectation of improving their fortunes."[9] The results would not always be promising, warned the Fredericton *Reporter*, for "we recommend, under the present circumstances, extreme caution to families entertaining a design to emigrate to that country [Australia]. To such we would say that many a difficulty, aye and many a *grave* lies between them and the realization of their wishes. For years to come any idea of the permanent and prosperous settlement of families in Australia must remain a problem. The mines have already robbed the soil of its natural rights and usages."[10] There were also warnings that the lifestyle of Australia might be detrimental to the welfare of Maritime youth, although a lively debate in the Saint John *Morning News* in 1852 between "Caution," "Justice," and "Ingram Sydney" over the climate, moral conduct and social progress of Australia tended to favour the antipodes.[11]

So also did some of the correspondence being sent back to the Maritimes by those who had already left. The *Novascotian* of 27 September 1852 reprinted from the *Cape Breton News* a letter in which a young man from Sydney, Nova Scotia, described his impressions of the Adelaide and Victoria diggings and the improvements he had seen in the country since his first visit in 1843. While he did not minimize the shortage of drinking water, poor health conditions, and potential for violence in the miners' camps, he nonetheless contributed to the popular conception of a better economic future should Maritimers immigrate to Australia:

> In these Colonies we may live cheaply — what is considered, in my native town (Sydney, Cape Breton) a very small sallary [sic], is quite enough to keep one comfortably here — This is chiefly owing to the fine climate here. There is no long six months winter to endure; and with very little interruption a man may work steadily throughout the whole year, which is a decided advantage. Besides, meat is seldom more than 3d per pound and generally from 1 1/2d. to 2d. Flour from 8 to l5 the ton; and clothing is by no means expensive. ... The gold of this country is said by many to be of much finer quality than that of California. The Diggers live in tents, and where there are thousands of

9   "State of Business," *Morning News*, 23 April 1852.
10 "The United States — Australia — New Brunswick," *The New Brunswick Reporter*, 9 July 1852.
11 "Correspondence. Australia!" *Morning Star* (Saint John), 21, 26, 31 May, 4, 9 June 1852.

all ages and both sexes thrown together, without order or law to protect them, you may conceive the state of society; however, hitherto things have been pretty orderly; and taking the population at Mount Alexander into consideration (45,000) crime has been light; but I do not think it can continue for a much longer period.[12]

James Robertson of Saint John, whose letters were published in the *Journal of the Royal Australian Historical Society* in March 1979, substantiated the Cape Bretoner's assessment. Expecting to make a few thousand pounds in a matter of years by servicing the miners as a sometime storekeeper, carpenter, shipowner, and investor, Robertson noted in November 1853: "I think there is no part of the globe to be compared to Australia — last winter was no colder here than the month of September is in New Brunswick." He outlined for his parents the amounts of money various Saint John people had already accumulated on the gold fields and by 1857 was urging his family in Saint John to immigrate to Australia because "this is distined [*sic*] to be one of the most productive farming Countries in the world."[13]

Nowhere is there a better sense of the conditions and prospects faced by Maritime Provinces adventurers in the goldfields, however, than in the private journals of those who tried to give shape to their impressions on a more sustained level than letter-writing. Of these, the unpublished "The Ballarat Riots" by Pax (Samuel Douglas Smith Huyghue of Saint John, New Brunswick) and "Pencillings On Sea and On Shore, or a Voyage to Australia" by Jacob Norton Crowell of Barrington, Nova Scotia, stand out because of the contrasting perspectives from which they are written. Of the two men, Huyghue was by far the more artistically-inclined and sophisticated in background and he narrates his account from the viewpoint of a gentleman and a government employee. Born in Charlottetown, Prince Edward Island in 1817, the son of Lieutenant Samuel Huyghue of the 60th Regiment of the Foot, he grew up in Saint John where his father was a half-pay officer, barrack master, and Head of the War Department. After receiving a classical education, Huyghue began to publish poetry in the Halifax *Morning Post* in 1840-41 under the pseudonym "Eugene," and between October 1841 and January 1843 he published poetry, fiction, and an essay on insect life in *The Amaranth* of Saint John. His novel, *Argimou. A Legend of the Micmac*, was serialized in *The Amaranth* between May and September 1842, and in 1847 was republished in book form. The first novel written by a Canadian to describe the 1755 expulsion of the Acadians, it was also one of the first fictions written in Canada to deplore the cultural deracination of the native

---

12 "Interesting From Australia," *Novascotian*, 27 September 1852.

13 Graeme Wynn, "Life on the Goldfields. Fifteen Letters. 1853-1861," *Journal of the Royal Australian Historical Society* (March 1979), pp. 4-5.

peoples as they were pushed toward economic and social assimilation by European settlement. "We are the sole and only cause of their overwhelming misery, their gradual extinction," notes the narrator at the beginning of the novel, and in the succeeding chapters he compares the virtues of natural life, "unrestrained by penal codes, or chains, or strong dungeons," with the hypocrisy and self serving demeanour of western civilization.[14] Huyghue's primitivist stance was romantic, but his knowledge of the Micmac and Malecite was always to be informed by first hand contact, by a scholarly study of their customs and culture (as demonstrated by an exhibition that he organized in the Mechanics' Institute of Saint John in 1842), and by his living amongst them from 1843 to 1845 as a commissary agent for the Boundary Commission surveying and marking the line between Maine, Quebec and New Brunswick. His accounts of that experience appeared in *Bentley's Miscellany* of London in 1849 and 1850 when Huyghue moved to England to try to develop his career as a writer, but the financial failure of his second romance of social conscience about native peoples, *The Nomads of the West, or, Ellen Clayton*, seems to have precipitated his decision to join the mass exodus from England to Australia. Arriving in Port Phillip on the "Lady Peel" on 4 February 1852, Huyghue joined the permanent staff of the civil service on 27 April 1853 and was appointed as a clerk in the Office of Mines at Ballarat on 27 August 1853.

The sense of morality that informed Huyghue's Canadian writing and made him a champion for social justice also enters his account of the Ballarat unrest, for although Huyghue was a government employee, a son of the garrison, and sympathetic to the young "cub" soldiers fighting for the first time, he was also critical of the bureaucratic policy and class insensitivity that had precipitated events leading to the Eureka Stockade. As he returns to his 1854 journals in 1879 and 1884, he is keenly conscious of the fact that "the miners, or diggers as they were then called, being unenfranchised, had no voice in the making of the laws, and were looked upon more as outcasts and vagabonds, than as worthy representatives of the intelligence and nation-founding energy of Great Britain, which they mostly were." He remarks on the incongruity of government attempts to make the members of the Gold Commission "aristocratic and exclusive" so that they went among "the mud-bespattered and blunt-spoken diggers" trucked out "in scraps of braid and gold lace, stamped with an air of authority, well-bred but lofty, and often redolent of perfume." Backed up by troops, these were the men, notes Huyghue, sent in by government to settle disputes or demand licenses. "The thing was out of all keeping with the surroundings," he adds. "It smacked too

---

14   'Eugene' [Samuel Douglas Smith Huyghue], *Armigou. A Legend of the Micmac* (1842; rpt. Sackville, 1977, 1979), pp. 92-93. See also Gwendolyn Davies, "Douglas Huyghue," *Dictionary of Canadian Biography*, XII (Toronto, 1990), pp. 462-63.

much of metropolitan and military grandeur for the votaries of the pick and spade, who were contemptuous of city ways."[15]

Elsewhere, Huyghue notes other administrative follies that exacerbated conditions in Ballarat in the fall of 1854. He is critical of the authorities' ill-judged preliminary acquittal of the hotelier Bentley for murder and the subsequent mishandling of events surrounding the torching of Bentley's Eureka Hotel; he is overwhelmed after the Eureka Stockade by the bureaucratic decision to resume armed searches for unlicensed miners, one of the causes of the diggers' original unrest; and he is both sympathetic to and critical of Sir Charles Hotham, a man who did not seek authority in Australia but who "having no faith in mankind generally and in colonists especially,...sought to embrace within his grasp the entire machinery of government; interfering most mischievously, and with a want of courtesy unknown to colonial tradition, with the ordinary departmental routine." While he describes Raffaello Carboni's book on the Eureka Stockade as being somewhat "wild," Huyghue nonetheless agrees with the Eureka Stockade leader "that the camp authorities, during this period were mere marionettes whose strings were pulled from Toorak," and he concludes his prose account with his own 1857 poem, "The Miner of the Stockade," in which he pays tribute to those archetypal figures who took a stand:

> Rear'd where the o'ertax'd nations give
> Their toil to fill the magnate's maw,
> He came to earn his bread and live
> Untrammel'd by patrician law.
> Hopeful he came — and nature spread
> Her treasures for her sturdy child:
> But misrule rais'd its baleful head
> And then outrang his war cry wild. —
> Stung into strife by outrage keen
> He was no rebel to his Queen.[16]

Throughout Douglas Huyghue's account of Ballarat, then, there is the sense of a man of strong moral conscience caught in a contradictory situation: a man who for four nights was armed and defended the government camp — a man who even as he writes laments the government's failure to maintain properly the graves of Eureka's slain military — nonetheless, a man who believes that the diggers had cause at Eureka and were often the victims of government stupidity. His situation as a Maritimer caught in a love-hate

---

15 "Pax" [Huyghue], "The Ballarat Riots, 1854," MS A1789, Mitchell Library, Sydney, Australia.

16 *Ibid.*, pp. 59, 52, 68-69.

relationship with Australia intensifies the outsider-insider theme informing his work, for as an 1857 diary entry on the back of his drawing "The Black Hill Ballarat 1857" in the State Library of Victoria makes clear, he has literally and symbolically never breathed such air as he has in Australia. "Nor do I think," he adds, "after having breathed it I could live on other air. This is a matter of regret for I cannot love this uncongenial land."[17] By the time that he had revised his journals of the 1850s, however, he has come to feel differently about "this uncongenial land." Nonetheless, the process, he noted, had been slow, for "My feelings of aversion to this country also were very strong. I could not shake off for many years after my arrival, a forlorn sense of exile under strange stars, and failed to recognize in the hard face of Australian nature, the face of a Mother."[18]

Huyghue's account of "The Ballarat Riots" therefore reflects not only his assessment of the events surrounding Eureka but also his gradual acclimatization to his adopted land. By the 1870s, time and experience had cast a certain romance over the past, he noted: "Somehow, I find myself clinging with a sort of fondness to the old picture; for there was an indescribable charm about the rough, unceremonious life of those early days, with their strong vitality and rapidly occurring incidents, — strange and exciting as those of a romance which enshrines it as an experience [*sic*] apart."[19] However, the end result of all experience, he adds, is conventionality. Whether he was thinking of the direction of his own life or of the subsequent conventional respectability of Eureka leaders like Peter Lalor and John Humffray, it is difficult to say, but a reading of Huyghue's revised 1854 journals in "The Ballarat Riots" suggests that he never quite succumbed to conventionality himself. Behind the fast-clipped pace, visual description, and levels of literary allusion in the account, there lurks still the persona of a moral man writing, whether it be in novels about native peoples in North America or in memoirs about diggers in Australia, so that social injustice and folly will be recognized.

There is nothing in Huyghue's account of Eureka to suggest that as he worked in the government camp as chief commissariat clerk in the 1850s he ever met other Maritime-Canadians who had migrated to the goldfields. Such is not the case when one turns to Jacob Norton Crowell's "Pencillings on Sea and on Shore, or a Voyage to Australia," a journal kept by the young seaman for three years and five months from the time he left Barrington, Nova Scotia, in June 1852 until he returned to Nova Scotia from the goldfields of Ballarat on 10 December 1855. Throughout Crowell's account the reader is aware of

---

17   Samuel Douglas Smith Huyghue, "The Black Hill Ballarat 1857," H25 190 *verso*, State Library of Victoria (Pictorial Section), Melbourne.

18   "Pax" [Huyghue], "The Ballarat Riots," p. 1.

19   *Ibid.*, p. 2.

the community sense of Maritime-Canadians as they embarked on the gold rush. Crowell and his Doane, Sargent, and Coffin relatives bought the 111 ton brigantine "Sebim" from Captain Warren Doane in order to sail to Ballarat, and they often pitched camp beside Maritimers and fellow Wesleyans on the goldfields. Crowell's journal is punctuated by news about recently arrived Maritime ships, incoming Barrington mail, welcome Halifax newspapers, the sale of Sam Slick books at a goldfields auction, and deaths at home and in the camp. Nova Scotian deaths fill Crowell with a sense of loss and, along with the lawlessness and post-Eureka politics that he witnesses, convince him on 9 July 1855 that he must return to his native land:

> I have concluded if all is well to leave this country and turn my steps homeward, and if I live I may be in Nova Scotia by the middle of November. I expect to leave in the Marco Polo about the 21st of this month.... I have not come to the determination of leaving for home hastily, but after a good deal of deliberation on the subject.... Thus believing that all is for the best, I am willing to leave this land of gold for one that is cold, sterile, and unproductive. There however there is some little happiness to be enjoyed among friends and I trust I shall be returned once more to them.[20]

Crowell's journal has a moralistic dimension to it absent from Huyghue's account, for the young Wesleyan was active in trying to stamp out alcohol on the goldfields and he yearned that "my native home, my country, be preserved" from the blight of an alcohol funded economy. This moralism extended into Crowell's politics, for he was disgusted after the Eureka Stockade uprising at the "Impious folly" of awarding Peter Lalor heroic status, and he remained loyal to Governor Sir Charles Hotham, who had once stopped by Mrs. Joseph Doane's Wesleyan Sabbath School and talked to the diggers. Crowell's viewing of the Eureka dead — "their bodies mangled with wounds and besmeared with dirt and gore, their faces set in the rigid expression of dying and maddening pain" — made an indelible impression on him and reinforced the conservatism of his politics. Yet even this gentle, religious man confessed to himself that "There is no doubt of the fact, we all feel that there is grievances that need to be redressed, and reforms are wanting in the government." Although he felt that "we should never have taken up arms when agitation and the voice of the people had not been properly heard," he nevertheless predicted from the experience of Eureka that "One thing is evident to the mind of the calm and careful observer of these

---

20 Jacob Norton Crowell, "Pencillings on Sea and on Shore, or a Voyage to Australia" [Journal of a Digger], Evelyn Richardson Papers, MG 1, vol. 1419, File 1, Item A, p. 128, PANS. See also Evelyn Richardson, *A Voyage to Australia* (Halifax, 1972).

ferments that the time *will* come when these colonies will no longer be under British Rule, but when another nation will hoist her standard and claim the respect due it from the various nations of the earth, and this be the Seagirt Continent of Australia."[21]

In analyzing the events of Eureka, Crowell does not have the political overview and sense of context that informs Huyghue's account, but he brings to his journal about the Ballarat goldfields a sense of immediacy, of lived experience, lacking in his more educated countryman's assessment. Crowell describes the blood spilt, feels the effects of the Tipperary raiders who threaten his claim, huddles in the rain and the cold, and notices first-hand with outrage the brutality directed at the Chinese diggers. He is a sensitive man who reads Hawthorne's *Twice-Told-Tales*, Cowper's works, and Emerson's discourses in his tent at night, and although his journal lacks the rhetorical polish and pacing of Huyghue's account, it occasionally breaks into lyrical descriptions of "fleecy clouds" or "the Sun in majestic splendour."[22] Moreover, there is a spontaneity of style about Crowell's descriptions lacking in Huyghue's more reflective retrospective account. On 4 December 1854 he outlines in unvarnished simple sentences the events of the Eureka Stockade the day before, "the ever memorable 3rd of December 1854 in the annals of Ballarat,"[23] culminating in his visit to the field of battle at nine o'clock and his description of the dead and wounded. By contrast, Huyghue sets his scene ("A hot wind had been blowing for two days"), heightens his pace ("the plot thickens too rapidly"), narrates self-consciously ("we will now recover the thread of our narration") and builds toward conflict ("three quarters of an hour.... This was immediately succeeded.... Now an outburst of flame...irregular firing continued for a time then dwindled away and ceased"). Yet in spite of the more narrative-oriented, almost novelistic demeanour of Huyghue's account, the impact of death affects him as honestly and as indelibly as it does Crowell. His viewing of the slain of both sides — the Eureka Stockade dead with "their faces ghastly and passion-distorted and their eyes staring with stony fixedness, and, in some instances, with their arms upraised, and fingers bent as though grasping a weapon in the death struggle" — moves him deeply, as does the plight of a small dog that faithfully accompanies the corpse of its master to the camp, ignorant, notes Huyghue, "either of Cross or Crown."[24]

For Huyghue, Eureka was to be a preoccupation for the rest of his life. He sent an early account of the events and a piece of the Southern Cross flag to his Melbourne friend, Reynell Eveleigh Johns, shortly after Eureka; his

---

21   Crowell, "Pencillings on Sea and on Shore", pp. 129-30, 120-21, 100, 101.

22   *Ibid.*, p. 108.

23   *Ibid.*, p. 99.

24   Huyghue, "The Ballarat Riots," pp. 3, 6, 14, 23, 32-33.

sketches and watercolours of Ballarat and Eureka are now in the collections of the La Trobe Library, the National Library of Australia, and the Ballarat Fine Arts Gallery and have been reproduced in a number of books, including William B. Wither's *The History of Ballarat* (1870), Alan McCulloch's *Artists of the Australian Goldrush* (1977), and Richard Butler's *Eureka Stockade* (1983); and in the 1870s and 1880s Huyghue revised his journals of the 1850s written when he was at Ballarat. He continued in the civil service in Ballarat, Graytown, and Melbourne until 1878 when he retired on a pension of £195 per year.[25] The diaries of Reynell Eveleigh Johns in the La Trobe Library substantiate an active literary, philosophical, and scientific correspondence between the two men from the 1850s until Huyghue's death in Melbourne in 1891 and reveal that Huyghue was current with such New Brunswick events as the 1877 great fire of Saint John (in which his parents lost all their property). At some point before 1873, he was joined in Australia by his unmarried sister, Emma Sophia Huyghue, who died in South Yarra in 1901.[26]

What of the other Maritimers who came to Ballarat? Unlike Huyghue, Jacob Norton Crowell did reach the Maritime Provinces again in 1855. He returned to his original occupation as a mariner and two years later was killed in a seafaring accident in Savannah, Georgia. His journal was given to a relative and exists now in typescript form in the Public Archives of Nova Scotia.[27] Some of his Barrington comrades who sailed with him on the "Sebim" to Australia also returned. Seth Doane worked in New Zealand on coal barges after leaving Australia and in 1873 made his way back to Barrington. In 1906 his nephew recalled: "He told me many yarns about his life in Australia and New Zealand. When mining he had led a hard life — I mean hard labour, long hours — picking and shovelling in tiring positions, sometimes on hands and knees, at other times tossing gravel several feet above his head. Now here he is at home, almost 80 years old, with the same quiet way.... Is a clerk of the church, keeps hens, has small fruit trees...."[28]

Arnold ("Arny") Doane, teacher and musician, and Jacob Norton Crowell's tentmate and particular friend at Ballarat, took his goldfield money to England and enrolled in the Academy of Music in London. He returned to Halifax after graduation to open an academy of music there, and eventually went back to Barrington where he authored *The History of Barrington*

---

25 *Ibid.*, p. 33.

26 MS 10075, Reynell Eveleigh Johns Papers, La Trobe Library, Melbourne, 4 June 1878; Emma S. Huyghue, Index to Probates 1900-1909, Hazel-Ryan, Victoria Public Record Office, 3340, Reel 6, Series 80, No. 862, Melbourne.

27 Evelyn M. Richardson published Crowell's description of his sea voyage to Australia as *A Voyage To Australia* (Halifax, 1972).

28 "Journal of a Digger," MS 1, vol. 1419, pp. 126-27, Evelyn Richardson Papers, PANS.

Township. Arthur Doane and Daniel Sargent returned, the latter marrying the sister of Sir John Thompson, Prime Minister of Canada, and becoming a prosperous Barrington merchant.[29]

Joseph Doane remained in Ballarat to become a leading architect, town councillor, and mayor. He designed at least eight Wesleyan churches in the Ballarat-Bendigo area, returned home to Barrington for a visit in 1875, and died in Melbourne in 1901.[30] Although memories of the great Australian goldrush experience remain in Barrington families to this day, those who sailed on the "Sebim" do not seem to have acquired the wealth of the two Prince Edward Islanders recorded in Crowell's diary or of James Robertson of Saint John who re-established himself in New Zealand with the money he had made from servicing the Ballarat goldfields.

For many Maritimers, as the Fredericton *Reporter* predicted, the Ballarat experience meant the grave. Huyghue, Robertson, and Crowell, say nothing of Robert Julien, the Nova Scotian who died at the Eureka Stockade or, for that matter, of Lieutenant Charles Ross, the Torontonian who also died at the Stockade and who reputedly designed the Southern Cross flag. Two of the three Barrington women on the expedition did not survive, and Crowell never forgot the loss of his cousin, Peter Coffin, who died of dysentery on the goldfields. For those Maritimers who did survive, however, Ballarat was clearly an experience that influenced the rest of their lives. "I can say that I am not disposed to regret that I have travelled so far," notes Jacob Norton Crowell at the end of his journal in 1855, "nor that I have passed through so many varieties of change — I have learned some useful and valuable lessons and think I am a *little wiser* for my pains." [31]

---

29 *Ibid.*, p. 128.

30 *Ibid.*, p. 127. See also *Reporter* (Halifax), 15 September 1864.

31 Crowell, "Pencillings on Sea and On Shore," p. 136.

James DeMille's *The Dodge Club*
and The Tradition of Nineteenth-Century
American Travel Literature

In Mark Twain's *The Innocents Abroad*, the passengers on the cruise ship
"Quaker City" gather in the saloon every night after prayers to write
"diligently in their journals" for "two or three hours." However, their
overwhelming desire to describe their travels is short-lived, notes Twain, and
he is "morally certain that not ten of the party can show twenty pages of
journal for the succeeding 20,000 miles of voyaging."[1]

Twain's personal attempt to keep a record of "the succeeding 20,000 miles
of voyaging" was more successful. Commissioned by the *Daily Alta
California* to write an account of the "Quaker City" excursion, Twain
subsequently reorganized his newspaper letters into *The Innocents Abroad*. In
doing so, he was appealing to a popular taste, for as increasing numbers of
American tourists crossed the Atlantic in the nineteenth century,[2] they sought
the observations and advice of their countrymen who had travelled to Europe
before them. Authors as established as Washington Irving, Nathaniel
Hawthorne, Ralph Waldo Emerson and William Dean Howells had preceded
Twain in turning their literary skills to descriptions of Old World travel and
culture, while professional tourists like Bayard Taylor and George Hilliard
produced formula travelogues to meet the public's demand for
comprehensive itineraries and background information.

By the time Twain published *The Innocents Abroad* in 1869, the American
travel book had undergone a number of transformations in style and content.
The travelogue of the 1840s had generally been an unimaginative affair
endorsing a grand tour of English and Continental landmarks. Its successor in
the 1850s tended to be somewhat more sentimental and varied in tone,
interspersing a wealth of travel information with personal essays on art,
architecture, and culture.[3] By the 1860s, however, the world of the American
travel book had again changed. Rapid-moving travellers eager to get the most
value for their tourist dollar demanded fact-filled, descriptive itineraries,
while a new generation of educated and sophisticated travellers called for
more exotic and far-flung destinations than had hitherto been popular.[4]
Responding to these interests and to a spirit of scepticism born of America's

---

1   Samuel Clemens [Mark Twain], *The Innocents Abroad or the New Pilgrim's Progress* (New
    York, 1966), p. 32.

2   Williard Thorp, *Literary History of the United States* (New York, 1973), p. 827.

3   Paul Baker, *The Fortunate Pilgrims* (Cambridge, 1964), p. 4, and Thorp, *Literary History*, p.
    831.

4   Thorp, *Literary History*, pp. 831-32.

growing commitment to scientific and technological values, the divisive effects of the Civil War, and increased travel abroad, a number of travel book writers turned to satire, caricature, and burlesque as a way of imaginatively expressing Americans' rapidly changing perception of themselves in both the United States and the broader world. Casting an irreverent eye on their countrymen as well as on Europeans, these authors often straddled the border between documentary and fiction, creating out of the traditional travel book a work which was as entertaining as it was enlightening.

Not least among the writers of the 1860s who contributed to the evolvement of the travelogue genre was a Canadian, James DeMille. Like Mark Twain, DeMille detected the sportive possibilities of the travelogue form, and in 1867 transformed his notes on a tour of France and Italy into the comic work, *The Dodge Club; Or, Italy In MDCCCLIX.* First serialized in *Harper's New Monthly Magazine* from March to October 1867, *The Dodge Club* was eventually published by Harper's in book form in 1869. Like Twain's *The Innocents Abroad* issued in the same year, *The Dodge Club* adopted a travelogue format while appealing to a broader readership. So popular was the book that it was described in its day as being "the fashionable subject of conversation in all circles of society," and none were said to enjoy its "crisp fun" more than the Americans, the people "whose little foibles and whims and caprices, the author intended to satirize."[5] However, the book's fun was due as much to its comic reversal of travelogue conventions as to its ironic portrait of American type figures abroad, and DeMille, like Twain, did much to turn the formula tour book of mid-century into a spirited and sometimes irreverent treatment of national shibboleths and national identities alike.

To explain the significant change in the travel genre represented by *The Dodge Club* and *The Innocents Abroad,* one need only turn to a traditional travelogue of mid-century, George Hilliard's *Six Months In Italy* published in 1853. Hilliard's was an ideal book for American tourists going abroad, for it combined a wealth of detail with a fellow countryman's understanding of American expectations. While the author does not analyze the confrontation between American and European values, he does confirm for Americans the desirability of their way of life. He notes that the selectman of New England has a more fruitful existence than does the Archduchess of Parma, and he concludes his tour with the smug notation that "the American does not see Italy aright who does not find there fresh cause of gratitude for having been born where he was...." Thus, his warning that "we travel to little purpose if we carry with us the standard which is formed at home" is ironically undercut

5   George Stewart, "Professeur James DeMille," in *"Scrapbook" Contenant Divers Souvenirs Personnels du Canada* by Compte de Premio-Real (Quebec, 1880), p. 182.

in the book by his own spirited affirmation that America is the land of the blessed.[6]

Hilliard's stated purpose in writing *Six Months In Italy* was to provide "hints and suggestions"[7] for the American travelling to that country, but inadvertently he says almost as much about America in the 1850s as he does about Italy. His typical American traveller is a "rapid" one demanding full value for the time and money he is devoting to his trip abroad, and Hilliard therefore feels it necessary to present a clear outline of what is worth seeing and the length of time it will take to see it. Thus, Parma receives a day in Hilliard's tour and Bologna is dismissed as requiring "more days than I had hours at command." Renunciation is one of Hilliard's travel philosophies, and the book proffers the advice: "choose what seems most interesting, and let the rest go."[8]

The itinerary Hilliard suggests is the conventional one of Lake Como, Milan, Venice, Florence, and Rome, although side excursions to places of architectural or historical interest are included for those with time for extra travelling. What strikes the modern reader most forcibly about this programme of travel is Hilliard's tendency to present everything in terms of its American counterpart. He does not discuss the architecture of Pompeii without comparing it to that of New England, nor does he describe a Raphael fresco without ruminating on its inability to capture the moral fervour of those who died at Bunker Hill. In short, although Hilliard can range over the world of Italian art, architecture, and music, and can descant in the language of Burkean sublimity on the beauty of the Bernese Alps, he is unable to divorce himself from the predilections and attitudes of his countrymen. These attitudes include America's admiration for industrialization and technology as manifestations of a nation's progressiveness and energy, and Hilliard clearly finds himself in contradictory circumstances as he praises Italy's architectural and historical heritage on one hand and America's scientific and industrial initiative on the other.

Nowhere is Hilliard's dilemma better illustrated than in his section on Venice, for he finds the city as beautiful as a "fairy pageant" and appreciates its romantic and original qualities. Yet Hilliard's progressive eye also detects the "decaying fortunes" and "unresisted dilapidation" of the great Italian city, and it is only by focusing on Venice's railroad as a symbol of reconciliation between the "old fields" and the "new corn" that he is able to accommodate himself to the conflict between material and cultural standards that the city suggests:

6   George Hilliard, *Six Months in Italy* (Boston, 1853), pp. 96, 230, 452.

7   *Ibid.*, Preface.

8   *Ibid.*, p. 100.

The railway not only connects Venice with the mainland, but the past and the future. It is an ennobling thought that the spirit of man is ever young, and that if it has ceased to speak in cathedrals and campaniles, it is yet vocal in railways, tubular bridges and magnetic telegraphs...and from the teeming brain of man there springs in one age a gondola, in another, a steamer; at one period, a Cologne Cathedral, at another, a Menai Bridge. Let us be thankful that we, who are now alive, have both the "old fields" and the "new corn."[9]

With its blend of personal opinion and solid travel information, Hilliard's *Six Months In Italy* is typical of the majority of travel books published in the United States between 1840 and 1860. Appealing to a touring public of at least 30,000 people annually,[10] Hilliard's work went into 21 editions and for many years enjoyed a secure place in the nineteenth-century American travel market. Yet even in the 1850s there were travel books being written in the United States that were beginning to break away from the traditional, formulaic pattern of *Six Months In Italy* with its emphasis on itinerary and information. Such a book was James Jackson Jarves' *Parisian Sights and French Principles Seen Through American Spectacles* published in New York in 1855. A collection of comic essays on Parisian social life as seen from an American point of view, it was designed to entertain rather than to inform. With its breezy tone and its emphasis on "originals" instead of fully developed characters, *Parisian Sights* in many ways anticipated James DeMille's *The Dodge Club* and Mark Twain's *The Innocents Abroad* to be published a decade later.

From the opening pages, neither DeMille's nor Twain's work claims to satisfy the demands of the traditional travel guide. Twain's preface to the "Quaker City" voyage begins with the provocative statement that the book is merely "a record of a picnic." It goes on to suggest that the design of *The Innocents Abroad or the New Pilgrim's Progress: Being Some Account of the Steamship "Quaker City's" Pleasure Excursion to Europe and the Holy Land* is to show the reader

> . . . how he would be likely to see Europe and the East if he looked at them with his own eyes instead of the eyes of those who travelled in those countries before him. I make small pretence of showing anyone how he *ought* to look at objects of interest beyond the sea — other books do that, and, therefore, even if I were competent to do it, there is no need.[11]

---

9   *Ibid.*, pp. 38, 87.

10   Baker, *The Fortunate Pilgrims*, p. 3.

11   Clemens, *The Innocents Abroad*, p. 15.

In such a statement, the Twain persona divorces himself from popular travel guides like Hilliard's and defines his role as that of a surrogate eye. As he boards the "Quaker City" with the ministers, professors, and families who make up the excursion, the narrator recognizes himself as part of the great middle class exodus to Europe that characterizes his age:

> Everybody was going to Europe — I, too, was going to Europe. Everybody was going to the famous Paris Exposition - I too, was going to the Paris Exposition. The steamship lines were carrying Americans out of the various ports of the country at the rate of four or five thousand a week in the aggregate. If I met a dozen individuals during that month who were not going to Europe shortly, I have no distinct remembrance of it now.[12]

The Americans described in this passage are the rapid travellers for whom Hilliard wrote — the tourists attracted in the thousands to Paris's Exposition or London's Crystal Palace. Thus, the "Quaker City" excursion of which Twain's narrator is a member is yet another example of America's nineteenth-century penchant for fast, comprehensive travel, for the ship's passengers seem typical of their time and their nation in wanting to visit the Azores, France, Italy, Greece, the Mediterranean, and the Holy Land, all within the brief compass of five months.

In spite of the persona's claim to be a surrogate eye for the passengers of the "Quaker City," he is spiritually the antithesis of the mundane middle class Americans with whom he is travelling. This puts him in an ideal position to be a satirist as well as an observer, and the reader finds the Twain persona assuming a variety of chameleon-like poses as he pokes fun at America, Europe, his fellow pilgrims, and himself. At once subject and object of the action, he is at the dramatic centre of the book in a way the Hilliard narrator is not. With wit, irony, irreverence, and burlesque as his weapons, he exposes the clown and the circus lurking beneath the surface of the journeyer and the journey respectively.

Twain partly exaggerates the conventions of the traditional travelogue to mock the genre, but he also remains true to elements of the parent form as a way of providing a formal structure for his work. In this sense, *The Innocents Abroad* satisfies what James Cox has called the "double vision" underlying burlesque,[13] for the Twain narrative functions successfully as a travelogue while it also channels the author's indignation and disillusionment into laughter. Thus, it is perfectly in character with burlesque conventions that the narrator not only visits the great art masterpieces of Europe as part of his

---

12   *Ibid.*, p. 24.

13   James Cox, *Mark Twain: The Fate of Humour* (Princeton, 1966), p. 44.

travel education but also mocks the self-consciousness of the exercise with exaggerated and irreverent comments:

> We have seen thirteen thousand St. Jeromes, and twenty-two thousand St. Marks, and sixteen thousand St. Sebastians, and four millions of assorted monks, undesignated, and we feel encouraged to believe that when we have seen some more of these various pictures and had a larger experience, we shall begin to take an absorbing interest in them like our cultivated countrymen from *Amerique*.[14]

Here, the Twain narrator not only exposes his own (and America's) uneasy confrontation with Europe's Catholic past, but also ridicules the pretentiousness of American travellers who go from picture to picture rhapsodizing over the "sublimity of conception" that the travelogues have schooled them to expect. Twain tends to be cynical about the effect of travelogues on the responses of unthinking American tourists, noting tartly that his fellow pilgrims may return from the "Quaker City" voyage able to "tell of Palestine, when they get home, not as it appeared to *them*, but as it appeared to Thompson and Robinson and Grimes —with the tints varied to suit each pilgrim's creed.[15]

Yet the Twain persona is himself not free of the prejudices and biases which his American background and reading have fostered, for there are long passages in *The Innocents Abroad* in which Twain praises the American way of life. Discoursing on the economic and spiritual poverty of modern Italy, he urges Italians to adopt his own nation's virtues of enterprise, self-reliance, and noble endeavour, a kind of American self image that DeMille satirizes through his Yankee Senator figure in *The Dodge Club*. Thus, there is a problem as the reader tries to relate to the Twain persona, for the persona may be unreliable. Twisting and turning throughout the book, he is at one moment the target of satire and at the next moment the agent of it. Portrayed as a man who covers his eyes with his hands to protect his innocence, he is also shown as irrepressibly peeking through his fingers. Thus, he is an experienced narrator in spite of himself — a man who may desire illusions but has none.

Although Bret Harte was to claim that the days of sentimental journeyings were over with the publication of *The Innocents Abroad*, *The Dodge Club In Italy* in its own way reinforced the "brickbats on stained-glass windows"[16] syndrome associated with Twain's energetic exposure of America's travel foibles. A fun-filled parody of travelogue conventions in addition to being a

---

14   Clemens, *The Innocents Abroad*, p. 171.

15   *Ibid.*, pp. 137, 369.

16   Foster Rhea Dulles, *Americans Abroad: Two Centuries of European Travel* (Ann Arbor, 1964), p. 109.

satire on American travel behaviour, *The Dodge Club* lacks the engaging central presence of Twain's irascible narrator. Whether sentimentally weeping over the grave of Adam in the Holy Land ("Noble old man — he did not live to see me — he did not live to see his child"), facetiously describing Venice's graceful gondolas as old "scows," or impishly watching the cancan ("I placed my hands before my face for very shame...but I looked through my fingers"), the Twain narrator is always a quicksilver and irreverent presence unifying *The Innocents Abroad.*[17]

The omniscient author who narrates the events of *The Dodge Club* is much less dramatic than is Twain's persona, but he is nonetheless a personable fellow who occasionally forsakes his duty as an objective chronicler of events to discuss the style or progress of the narrative with the reader: "There — I flatter myself that in the way of description it would not be easy to beat the above. I just throw it off as my friend Titmarsh, poor fellow, once said, to show what I could do if I tried. I have decided not to put punctuation marks there, but rather to let each reader supply them for himself."[18] By occasionally intruding into the book in this vein, the DeMille narrator brings a "novel in process" quality to *The Dodge Club* that undercuts its formal journey structure and contributes to the parody of the travelogue genre taking place in the book. DeMille's interpolations of this kind are limited in number, so they do not distract from the Dodge Club's adventures. Nonetheless, there are sections like Chapter XXXVII where the author clearly has fun at the expense of the travel reader's expectations. Under the headings, "Rome — Ancient History," "Topography," and "Remarks On Art," the narrator outlines his plan for a "thoroughly exhaustive"[19] chapter on the Eternal City, but he argues that the inclusion of such typical travelogue material has absolutely nothing to do with the main story and therefore will be excluded. Pretending that he will publish the definitive book on the subject after he has completed such mock scholarly endeavours as "The Toads of Maine" and the "Report of the Kennebunkport, Maine, United Congregational Ladies' Benevolent City Missionary and Mariners' Friend Society," the narrator resumes the Dodge Club tales, abandoning all pretence of providing a serious travelogue description of Rome and its environs. It is on occasions like this that the reader can detect DeMille's impish treatment of the journey format and his determination to adhere to travelogue conventions only as they suit his comic design.

If the author's self-conscious address to the reader occasionally turns the travel dimension of the book topsy-turvy, the presence of the Dodge Club itself adds a spirited and unorthodox element to DeMille's account.

---

17   Clemens, *The Innocents Abroad*, pp. 99, 166, 409.

18   James DeMille, *The Dodge Club; Or, Italy in MDCCCLIX* (New York, 1869), p. 42.

19   *Ibid.*, p. 88.

Organized around the group's desire "to dodge all humbugs and swindles, which make travelling so expensive"[20] in Europe, the Dodge Club consists of five representative American male travellers. Buttons and Dick Whifletree are resourceful young men who approach Europe's eccentricities with Yankee "cuteness" rather than with the mock innocence of Twain's narrator. On the other Hand, their companions, Senator Jones, Dr. Snakeroot, and Mr. Figgs are gull figures who are forever being extricated from the situations in which their cultural naivete has embroiled them. Together, the five ramble through France and Italy brashly announcing their Americanness wherever they go, and, in so doing, become agents and targets of DeMille's gentle satire on American nationalism and boosterism.

The most pronouncedly American of DeMille's creations in *The Dodge Club* is Senator Jones of Massachusetts, a literary offspring of Sam Slick, the fast-talking Yankee pedlar made famous by Thomas Chandler Haliburton in *The Clockmaker*.[21] Like Sam, the Senator is an exponent of his country's "go-ahead" tendencies, describing at length America's industrial initiative, financial astuteness, and scientific expertise. These attitudes, combined with his colourful vocabulary, his fanatical loyalty to Yankee Doodle-ism, and his ring-tailed roarer proclivities, all combine to make the Senator a caricature of a "typical" Yankee industrialist and republican. While DeMille does not fail to show the generous side of the American character through Jones, there is no doubt that the author is using the lanky Senator to satirize the parochialism, aggressiveness, and aesthetic insensitivity of an American type travelling abroad:

> These I-talians air a singular people. They're deficient. They're wanting in the leading element of the age. They haven't got any idee of the principle of progress. They don't understand trade. There's where they miss it. What's the use of handorgans? What's the use of dancers? What's the use of statoos, whether plaster images or marble sculptoor? Can they clear forests or build up states? No, Sir: and therefore I say that this Italian nation will never be wuth a cuss until they are inoculated with the spirit of Seventy-six, the principles of the Pilgrim Fathers, and the doctrines of the Revolution.[22]

---

20 *Ibid.*, p.6.

21 Thomas Chandler Haliburton's *The Clockmaker* first appeared in book form in 1836 and subsequently went into many editions in Great Britain and the United States. In his 1880 article, "Professeur James DeMille," George Stewart notes that "The Maritime Provinces enjoy the unusual reputation of having furnished two of the most striking portraitures of the 'Yankee' — Judge Haliburton's, whose 'Sam Slick' is the Yankee of the past, and James DeMille's, whose Yankee is the shrewd individual of the present day" (p. 183).

22 DeMille, *The Dodge Club*, p. 16

American cultural assumptions were something to which James DeMille could turn a detached and ironic eye, for although he knew the United States intimately from his studies and travels there, he was deeply rooted in his Maritime and Loyalist background. The son of Nathan DeMill,[23] a well known Saint John, New Brunswick, merchant and ship owner, he graduated from Horton Academy and Acadia College in Wolfville and in 1854 received a Master's degree from Brown University in Rhode Island. After an unsuccessful attempt at running a book and stationery business in Saint John, DeMille joined the faculty of Acadia in 1860 as a Professor of Classics. From Acadia he moved to Dalhousie University in 1865, holding the Professorship of History and Rhetoric there until his unexpected death in 1880. At that time, DeMille was being considered for the Chair of Rhetoric at Harvard and had completed the *Elements of Rhetoric*, a scholarly text which marked the culmination of seven years of research and writing. Fluent in Latin, Greek, Italian, and Hebrew, he was also interested in Sanskrit, Arabic, and Icelandic, and on occasion employed his facility with languages to introduce exotic dialects or phrases into novels like *A Strange Manuscript Found In A Copper Cylinder* or *The Dodge Club in Italy*.

DeMille's career as a popular novelist began as an attempt to liquidate debts incurred in running his Saint John book business in the late 1850s. However, the notebooks and records of DeMille's years at Brown University reveal that he had always had a comic and narrative turn of mind and was noted among his fellow students for his seemingly effortless ability to toss off caricatures, witty rhymes, and tall tales.[24] Thus, it is not surprising that DeMille was able to extract time from his busy teaching schedule at Acadia and Dalhousie to produce a series of clever adventure stories and melodramatic historical romances appealing to a mass reading audience, for, in the words of Archibald MacMechan, DeMille had the facility to shake "his novels out of his sleeve."[25] It is also not surprising that DeMille deliberately slanted his style, content, and characterization to suit American public taste and East Coast publishing interests, for with an eye to his debts and the saleability of his books, he clearly discerned America to be a more lucrative and receptive market than Canada. For this reason, most of DeMille's fiction first appeared with New York and Boston publishing houses and, for this reason, he seemed to many in his own time to be a part of the American

---

23 DeMille's family always spelled the name without an 'e' on the end. Throughout his life, DeMille used both spellings, but he always published his fiction under "DeMille."

24 The DeMille Papers are lodged in the Dalhousie University Archives in Halifax. For a full discussion of DeMille, see: Patricia Monk, *The Gilded Beaver: An Introduction to the Life and Work of James DeMille* (Toronto, 1990).

25 Archibald MacMechan to Lawrence Burpee, 28 February 1924, James DeMille Papers, Dalhousie University Archives.

literary mainstream rather than the Canadian one. Nonetheless, DeMille clearly thought of himself as a Canadian, and the ironic tone of a book like *The Dodge Club* suggests the sense of detachment with which he approached American national characteristics.

Although *The Dodge Club* appeared in 1867, it had as its genesis a trip to France and Italy which DeMille and his brother, Elisha, took in 1850-51. In the next decade, DeMille seems to have worked impressions of his continental journey into essay form, for 21 sketches of Rome and seven descriptions of Naples appeared in *The Christian Watchman* of St. John in 1860-61. It is during this period that DeMille supposedly detected the comic and fictional possibilities of his travel experiences, and his translation of these experiences into burlesque and satire therefore preceded Twain's attempt to do something similar with the "Quaker City" voyage of 1867. The question of influence raised in contemporary discussions of the two books[26] seems an unproductive avenue to follow, however, for clearly DeMille was in Halifax polishing his comic sketches for *Harper's New Monthly Magazine* at approximately the same time as Twain was at sea composing his "Quaker City" letters for the *Alta California*. What the similarity between the two books does suggest is the astuteness of the respective authors in sensing shifts in travelogue taste in the 1860s and their mutual sensitivity to publishers' demands for new and sprightly treatments of a tired form.

Given the fact that DeMille and Twain were working from common assumptions about the American travelling public and the potential of the travel book genre, it is interesting to note the somewhat different approaches they adopted in developing their material. By assuming a third person point of view, DeMille diffused among five characters and his narrator the satiric and comic observations that Twain was able to focus in one. The result is that *The Dodge Club* seems to lack the hard edge and singleness of purpose found in *The Innocents Abroad*, for no character in the DeMille book sustains interest in the way the Twain persona does. This occurs partly because DeMille envisages the club members as types — in some cases, even as caricatures — and partly because he intends action and not character to be the centre of his book. While people do have opinions in *The Dodge Club* and do in fact share the suspicion of European culture and admiration for American progressiveness found in the Twain narrator, they function in the book as

---

26   Lawrence Burpee, "Canadian Novels and Novelists," *The Sewanee Review* (October 1903), p. 393. An unidentified newspaper clipping of the period now found in the DeMille Papers at Dalhousie University also explores this question: "The latter [The Dodge Club] is a delightfully amusing bit of fiction in the manner of Mark Twain's 'Innocents Abroad,' published the same year but after DeMilles Book. It is highly improbable that Mr. Clemens got his idea from Professor DeMille, but certainly the Canadian writer could not have plagiarized the work of the American humorist. It was probably one of those literary coincidences with which we are all familiar."

lively representative forces acting out pre-ordained roles in the narrative rather than as fully developed acerbic voices designed to satisfy the reader's satiric sense.

DeMille's conception of *The Dodge Club* as a rambling, semi-picaresque travelogue is reinforced by the diversity of subject matter and approach he introduces into the club's travel pattern. Although in Chapter XXXVII the travelogue dimension of the book seems to be subverted by the narrative line, there are other occasions where DeMille includes letters, lists, and an article to the *New England Patriot* as ways of reinforcing his parody of American travellers and travelogues alike. Anticipating a theme that was to be central to Henry James's international novels, DeMille also presents a clash of cultures in several lively encounters between the club and the nationals they are visiting. One of the most memorable and dramatically effective of these is the scene in Rome between Senator Jones and La Cica in Chapter XLIII, an encounter which develops cleverly and ironically around the Senator's gauche misunderstanding of the Countess's social assumptions. A scene highly regarded in its time as a spoof on American parochialism and puritanism, the Senator-La Cica sequence was dramatized by the British actress Mrs. Scott Siddons and was performed in Halifax in 1879 with DeMille in the audience.

With its wide range of characters and approaches, it is sometimes difficult to discern the intended target of DeMille's spoofery and fun. At different times, the book seems to burlesque everything from American chauvinism and European degeneracy to travelogue conventions and the Dodge Club's ringtailed roarer escapades. Whatever the focus DeMille intended, *The Dodge Club* clearly lacks the impact that Twain achieved by consolidating burlesque, satire, and social commentary in the character of the narrator. Nonetheless, *The Dodge Club* often provides more lively reading than does *The Innocents Abroad*, for DeMille relied far more than did Twain on action, dialogue, conflict, and dramatic confrontation as means of elevating his work beyond the level of mere travelogue. One need only look at the ways in which Hilliard, Twain, and DeMille treat the traveller's obligatory visit to Pompeii to see how DeMille retains only enough of the travel form to suit his fictional purposes. Hilliard in *Six Months In Italy* factually describes the railway into Pompeii, the guides at the station, the composition of the ash that buried the city, the architecture of the houses, and the lusty paintings on the walls. Twain, on the other hand, combines sentimentalism with burlesque in his Pompeii sequence. At one moment railing at the city fathers of Pompeii for having ruts in their streets, the narrator is at the next moment mourning the fate of prisoners who were fettered to the wall as volcanic ash rained about them. However, as Daniel McKeithan points out in *Travelling With The Innocents Abroad*, one of Twain's main interests in the book is in provoking laughter.[27] Thus, a serious story of a soldier's nobility which Twain included in the *Alta California* letters is transformed into a throwaway soldier-policeman joke in *The Innocents Abroad*. It earns Twain an easy laugh, but it does so at the expense of something human and unstrained found in the author's original version.

The soldier joke is the kind of humour that one can also find in *The Dodge Club*, but DeMille skilfully integrates the Pompeii sequence into his narrative line. Focusing on the Senator's responses, the episode becomes a vehicle for dramatic exchange, for characterizing Senator Jones, and for revealing principles of Yankee utilitarianism. It is in his reaction to the story of the steadfast Roman soldier who would not forsake his post that the Senator and his pragmatism are seen in their most characteristic light:

> From the villa of Diomedes they went to the gate where the guardhouse is seen. Buttons told the story of the sentinel who died there on duty, embellishing it with a few new features of an original character.
>
> "Now that may be all very well," said the Senator, "but don't ask me to admire that chap, or the Roman army, or the system. It was all hollow. Why, don't you see the man was a blockhead? He hadn't sense enough to see that when the whole place was going to the dogs, it was no good stopping to guard it. He'd much better have cleared out and saved his precious life for the good of his country. Do you suppose a Yankee would act that way?"[28]

Typically, the Dodge Club leaves Pompeii shortly after this declaration and goes on to another tourist site and another adventure. As the group travels, the Senator continues to greet new places and shrines with irreverence and bombast, transforming scene after scene on the itinerary into a parody of American popular opinion and contributing to the general tone of levity that characterizes DeMille's work.

A tone of levity seems to be what the travel books of Jarves, Twain, and DeMille all have in common, and, in retrospect, these three men seem in the forefront of a group of writers destined to carry the American travel book in new directions after mid-century. Williard Thorp has noted in the *Literary History of The United States* that divisions and subdivisions of the travel genre continued to emerge in the last part of the nineteenth century, with the international novel being only one manifestation of the shifting form.[29] With more and more Americans flocking to Europe after 1850 — more than 30,000

27   Daniel M. McKeithan, *Travelling With The Innocents Abroad* (Norman, 1958), p. 81.

28   DeMille, *The Dodge Club*, p. 38.

29   Thorp, *Literary History of the United States*, p. 827.

per year just to Rome in the 1890s[30] — it is not surprising that new attitudes and new expectations should encourage changes in the genre. The conventional travelogue of the 1840s was destined to become the increasingly literary travel book of the late 1800s as growing numbers of Americans tested Ralph Waldo Emerson's dictum that "travelling is a fool's paradise."[31]

---

30   Baker, *The Fortunate Pilgrims*, p. 3.

31   Ralph Waldo Emerson, "Self-Reliance," in S. Bradley, R.C. Beatty, and E.H. Long, eds., *The American Tradition in Literature* (New York, 1961), p. 1084.

"A Past of Orchards":
Rural Change in Maritime Literature
Before Confederation

Wandering through the ruins of an old house by Cumberland Basin, the speaker of Douglas Lochhead's *Vigils & Mercies* sees "the scales of shingles go in their softening time," the "Glass gone," the "Frames wrenched out." "I rant," he notes, "to bring it back, alone, this telling, working, prayer-backed place." But the house stands "bare-strutted," a "Broken body with empty eyes" where "the dead have left their barn boots, their party shoes." Only the field remains, sloping down to where "the red bay holds." "Let me spend more nights, more days crouching, voiceless," proclaims the speaker, "confused by old prayers, no joy but the deep tremor within me. The rude limbs of lilacs pierce through leather. A sign? I would die. For a song. Give me words."[1]

Words can form a link, "can be like fires, flames around the heart"[2] in *Vigils & Mercies*, but they can do little to breathe life into a dead past. Agents of record, of memory, they struggle to impose meaning where meaning has disintegrated. The note of change sounded in the poems is both personal and social, a tentative exploration of human loss on several levels and an indirect reflection on the decline of rural life. Set in the same windswept expanse of Cumberland Basin as is Sir Charles G.D. Roberts' "Tantramar Revisited," *Vigils & Mercies* brings to fruition Roberts's fear that the "Hands of chance and change" will touch even here, "all I most have adored." A century separates the writing of the two poems, but in that period the "scattering houses stained with time" and the "orchards, meadows, and wheat" so admired by Roberts have ceased to be held in "darling illusion."[3] Now raped, kicked, and desecrated, this "old hack of a house" has become for Lochhead "a sign," "a song," a symbol of "the hallowed dead" and a "temple-cover" for his vigil. Nature lives with "tidal breath" and "sensuous curves" redolent with "so much inside us in the same condition." What is man-made, however, lies "dead," "the world's morgue," its "anatomy...unveiled."[4]

The note of rural change sounded by both Charles G.D. Roberts and Douglas Lochhead has a significant ring for anyone familiar with Raymond Williams's *The Country and the City*, Leo Marx's *The Machine in the*

---

1   Douglas Lochhead, "Vigils & Mercies," *The Antigonish Review*, 62-63 (Summer-Fall 1985), pp. 54, 55, 64. "A Past of Orchards" is found on p. 61.

2   *Ibid.*, p. 65.

3   Desmond Pacey, ed., *The Collected Poems of Sir Charles G.D. Roberts* (Wolfville, 1985), pp. 78-79.

4   Lochhead, *Vigils*, pp. 34, 55, 65.

Garden, Roderick Nash's *Wilderness and the American Mind*, or John F. Kasson's *Civilizing the Machine*. What is less familiar, perhaps, is the degree to which this theme entered Maritime literature in even its earliest, most formative stages. The clash between urban and rural values, between the economic aggressiveness of the city and the agrarian rhythms of the country, can be found not only in the poems of late Victorian scepticism but also in earlier works emanating from the eighteenth-century confrontation of progress and order. As early as 1789, a "Farmer from Cornwallis" had noted that a new journal from Halifax was beyond the ken of the ordinary Annapolis Valley worker because "cash in this country is quite out of use." Commercial centres of gravity lay not in rural landscapes but in urban areas like Halifax, and in the doggerel verses of this "honest Hibernian" farmer outlining the dilemma of a country man yearning for a city commodity, he revealed the pressures exerted on the old rural barter system by the insistence of the city on cold cash. Editor William Cochran's response to this poetic epistle from Cornwallis was to offer *The Nova-Scotia Magazine* (1789-92) to the farmer for a shipment of bluenose potatoes, adding as an ironic afterthought that he hoped the quality of the potatoes exceeded the quality of the verses.

The product of rural life himself, Cochran well understood the threat posed to a barter economy by the urban demand for money, and he no doubt sympathized with the dilemma of the common man who found the world's division into the privileged and the classless based on those who could afford to pay and those who could not: "It exceedingly pleas'd me, and made me inquire/ How I could obtain it; Why, answered the Squire/ You may have twelve a year, for the trifling expence/ Of four crowns, two shillings, and one single six-pence."[5] An Irishman by birth, and one who had originally immigrated to the New World because of his support for the American Revolutionary cause, Cochran may well have identified with the historical status of the "honest Hibernian" writing the poetic epistle from Cornwallis. Freed of the squirearchy in Ireland, the farmer seems to have come among the settled New England husbandmen of the Annapolis Valley and found a social structure of prosperous landowners and tenantry not dissimilar to that left behind. Certainly, the farmer's Irish presence in the established New England character of Cornwallis suggests the patterns of ethnic migration and change taking place in late eighteenth-century Nova Scotia, as does the reference in his poem to the threat posed to traditional religious authority by the introduction of itinerant Methodist preachers and their tracts into rural life: "I thought at first sight, 'twas a Methodist sermon./ The country, of late, being full of such vermin."

---

5   Farmer of Cornwallis, "Poetical Letter to the Editor of *The Nova-Scotia Magazine*," *The Nova-Scotia Magazine*, I (November 1789), p. 389.

Unchanging as one would think Nova Scotian rural life to be in 1789, a single vernacular poem suggests the very opposite. Church authority is being eroded, money has become an increasingly visible arbiter of class and comfort, and immigration is changing the traditional population-base of the settlement. Douglas Lochhead's "dead" who "have left their barn boots," and *The Nova-Scotia Magazine*'s Hibernian farmer from Cornwallis, might exist 200 years apart, but they share in their vulnerability to Roberts's "hands of chance and change" a common denominator that unifies the literature of eighteenth-century Maritime Canada with that of the twentieth. The difference lies, however, in the shift in emphasis and perspective that takes place over that 200 year period, for in "Tantramar Revisited" and in *Vigils & Mercies*, there is a sense of regret over what may have been lost, a feeling that something worth preserving may have disappeared. In the 1789 poetical epistle from "A Farmer from Cornwallis," on the other hand, there is none of Roberts's defensiveness about the winds of "chance and change." The farmer may be sceptical of the new Methodist vermin and chafing under the absence of "cash in the country," but he is yearning to read the "new magazine" from Halifax, reaching out to embrace the forces that will shatter his isolation and eventually make him part of the march of progress going on beyond the Valley.

The contrast in tone between the 1789 *Nova-Scotia Magazine* poem and the poems of Sir Charles G.D. Roberts and Douglas Lochhead is the contrast one also finds in reading Thomas McCulloch's 1821 *The Stepsure Letters* and in reading Stephen Leacock's 1912 *Sunshine Sketches of a Little Town*. In Leacock there is a regretful looking-back to Mariposa, a yearning for a town rich in human resources and the values of rural community. The "L'Envoi" at the end of the sketches presents a former Mariposan returning to his old haunts and discovering in true Thomas Wolfe fashion that "you can't go home again."[6] "No, don't bother to look at the reflection of your face in the window-pane," admonishes the narrator, "nobody could tell you now after all these years. Your face has changed in these long years of money-getting in the city."[7] The idealized small town basking in the golden sunshine must remain just that — an illusion bittersweet in memory and irretrievable from the course of time.

Although Leacock's *Sunshine Sketches of a Little Town* and his *Arcadian Adventures with the Idle Rich* (1914) are set in Ontario and the United States respectively, they say much about the literary reaction to rural change that had entered Canadian literature by 1900. As with Roberts's "Tantramar Revisited," there is a wistful process of mythologization taking place, a Brigadoon of the mind that creates a small town marked by friendship,

6   Thomas Wolfe, *Look Homeward, Angel* (New York, 1929).
7   Stephen Leacock, *Sunshine Sketches of a Little Town* (1912; rpt. Toronto, 1969), p. 152.

community activities, and a sense of common pride. Satire, when it does exist, is of the gentle Horatian variety found in Leacock's *Sunshine Sketches,* where the follies and foibles of human nature are held up to ridicule and create a loveable collection of eccentrics worthy of the town's romanticization.

How completely the pendulum had swung by the time of *Sunshine Sketches of a Little Town* is nowhere better illustrated than in a reading of Thomas McCulloch's *Mephibosheth Stepsure Letters* written for *The Acadian Recorder* from 1821 to 1823, or of *The Clockmaker* (1835) and *The Old Judge or Life in a Colony* (1849) written by McCulloch's successor, Thomas Chandler Haliburton. In both cases, the works are composed by authors who are deeply committed to the Maritime region in which they live, and the satire to which they resort is as forward-looking in intent as it is precise in tone. Whereas Roberts holds time in stasis and Leacock looks back to a halcyon era of youth, McCulloch and Haliburton write for the improvement and progressive change of their rural economies. Sam Slick borrows the phrase "Go Ahead" from Davy Crockett,[8] and Mephibosheth Stepsure consciously or unconsciously echoes Benjamin Franklin in his pronouncement: "Everyman who works for his neighbour knows time to be money."[9] Both axioms suggest practical advancement.

Thomas McCulloch turned to the Stepsure letters at a time when sweeping economic and social changes were taking place in rural Nova Scotian life. The Napoleonic Wars had created artificial markets, had escalated the timber trade, had generated local ship-building, and had provided farmers with guaranteed outlets for their crops. *The Mephibosheth Stepsure Letters* record this phenomenon, but record it at the historical moment when it is in a state of decline after the cessation of hostilities. "It has been, in our town," says Stepsure, "a time of general distress."[10] As has so often been the case in the history of Maritime literature, war proved to be the catalyst for a period of literary activity and social upheaval. In the assembly of type characters sketched by McCulloch's self-righteous persona, Mephibosheth Stepsure, there is ample evidence of the way in which the Jack Scorems and the Mr. Goslings of the community have been lured off their farms by the easy profits of a war-time economy:

> Jack was in debt, and known to be a good axeman; and just when he was beginning to clear up his new land, Mr. Ledger's tempting offers

---

8   V.L.O. Chittick, *Thomas Chandler Haliburton: A Study in Provincial Toryism* (1924; rpt. New York, 1966), pp. 375-76.

9   Thomas McCulloch, *The Mephiboseth Stepsure Letters,* ed. Gwendolyn Davies (Ottawa, 1990), p. 143.

10   *Ibid.,* p. 28.

interrupted the farming. He might jump into the woods in the morning, and at night return home two or three dollars richer. This was a prospect not to be despised by one who was in debt; and besides, wished to have his house and barn finished.[11]

It has been endemic in Maritime society to follow the promise of fast money. From privateering to fox farming, to rum running, to Atlantic Lotto, Maritimers have pursued the dream of freeing themselves from toil and making the fortune that will provide them with what McCulloch calls "tea and trumpery." Jack Scorem's is just one of many tales of decline and fall told by Stepsure to illustrate McCulloch's main thesis in the *Letters* — that hard work, prudence, faithfulness to the fields, family values, and religious piety all contribute to the stability, happiness, and prosperity of both individuals and communities. With a deviation from the norm, there is moral and economic disaster. With adherence to the norm, one enjoys the enviable position of Stepsure and his cohorts:

> Whoever looks at the soil of our township, would say that nature designed us to be a farming people; and, that every man who gives the ground fair play, will be able to live very snugly. Accordingly, my cousin Harrow, Saunders Scantocreesh, and a few others, who mind only their farms, have everything thriving about them; and whoever goes into their houses, is sure to find plenty and cheerfulness. Yet, though our soil is excellent, and farms very easily got, the most of our townsfolk would rather ride two days round the country to make a bargain, than give the ground one day's labour. Whether this proceeds from the waywardness of human nature, or, because being British subjects, we are born traders, I cannot tell.[12]

McCulloch was not alone in striking a warning note about the state of Nova Scotia agriculture and the short-sightedness of neglecting a mixed farming economy in the early years of the nineteenth century. Whether William Cochran's essays on farming in *The Nova-Scotia Magazine* in 1789, Lord Dalhousie's observations in his 1816-20 journal, Agricola's letters to *The Acadian Recorder* in 1818-19, or Joseph Howe's comments in the "Eastern" and "Western Rambles" a few years later, there was an acute consciousness on the part of observers that too many rural dwellers sought the pride of silk rather than the modesty of homespun.[13] However, whereas their essays often

---

11   *Ibid.*, p. 21.

12   *Ibid.*, p. 29.

13   W. See, "A Plan Of Liberal Education For The Youth Of Nova-Scotia, and the Sister Provinces in North-America," *The Nova-Scotia Magazine*, I (August 1789), pp. 105-06; 1

appealed to only a select audience, McCulloch's earthy, double-edged satire with its pawky and objectionably pompous narrator enraged, delighted, and fired vast numbers of the common newspaper-reading public when the letters began to circulate in *The Acadian Recorder* in 1821. "So true to fact were they," noted McCulloch's son, William, that

> in almost every part of the country the different characters were supposed to be recognized. No little indignation was expressed by those who thought themselves caricatured, and many were the efforts made to locate the audacious slanderer. A gentleman describing the effect of those letters in his own neighbourhood said "We looked with great anxiety for the arrival of *The Recorder*, and on its receipt used to assemble in the shop of Mr. _____ to hear 'Stepsure' read, and pick out the characters, and comment on their foibles, quite sure that they were among ourselves." Great was often the anger expressed, and threats uttered against the author if they could discover him.[14]

How successful McCulloch's *Mephibosheth Stepsure Letters* were in effecting reform is problematical, but as a reinforcement of literary convention, they had an important impact in heightening the contrast between city and country already introduced into Maritime literature in the eighteenth century by such writers as Henry Alline, "Pollio,"[15] and the "Farmer from Cornwallis." McCulloch showed, as would his successor Stephen Leacock, the destructive intrusion of urban values on rural life. Stepsure's town is no more successful than is Mariposa in its aping of the customs of the big city, and it is when Mr. Gosling's Polly goes to Halifax "to sell her turkeys and see the fashions" that a process of domestic disintegration begins that leads to "puddings and pies" of "mere dough."[16] "To be genteel in the country" notes Stepsure drily, "is attended with difficulties and losses of which you townsfolk can have no conception."[17]

McCulloch's letters paved the way psychologically and thematically for the later sketches of Thomas Chandler Haliburton, who as early as his 1823 and 1829 histories of Nova Scotia had begun to address the question of the

(September 1789), pp. 199-203; I (November 1789), pp. 364-66; Marjory Whitelaw, ed., *The Dalhousie Journals* (Ottawa, 1978); John Young, *The Letters of Agricola* (Halifax, 1822); Joseph Howe, *Western and Eastern Rambles: Travel Sketches of Nova Scotia*, ed. by M.G. Parks (Toronto, 1973).

14 William McCulloch, *Life of Thomas McCulloch, D.D.* (Truro, 1920), p. 73.

15 "Pollio" was a pseudonymous poet who published in *The Nova-Scotia Magazine* in 1789-90. In "Rural Happiness" (December 1789), he decried urban life and praised the beauties of his "native woods."

16 McCulloch, *The Mephibosheth Stepsure Letters*, pp. 8 and 13.

17 *Ibid.*, p. 13.

province's real nature.[18] No less concerned than McCulloch with Nova Scotians' desertion from the homespun,[19] Haliburton presented in his Stephen Richardson figure in *The Old Judge* a rural spokesman as traditional in his approach to the land as Mephibosheth Stepsure:

> "I don't pity you a morsel," said Stephen. "The best office for a farmer is being his own overseer, and the best fees those paid by his orchards and fields. There is nothing so mean in folks like you and me as office seeking, unless it is in wearing broadcloth instead of homespun, as if a man was above his business. Now look at me," and he rose up and stood erect; "I am six feet four in my stockings, when unravelled and bolt upright, and six feet five when stretched out on a bench; and, from the sole of my foot to the crown of my head, I am dressed in the produce of my own farm. I raised the flax and hackled it, and bred the sheep and sheared the wool that made the linen and the cloth that I wear. I am sort of proud of it, too; for a farmer, according to my idea of things, ought to be known by his dress, like an officer or a parson; and then, when folks see him, they'll know he ain't run up a bill at the shop, and ain't cutting a dash in things he han't paid for."[20]

However much Haliburton admired the Stephen Richardsons of the countryside, he responded more flexibly and perhaps more realistically than did McCulloch to the impact of social and technological change on the rural economy of the Maritimes. His Bluenose, he noted in the "Preface" to *The Old Judge*, was a man who

> is often found superintending the cultivation of a farm or building a vessel at the same time; and is not only able to catch and cure a cargo of fish, but to find his way with it to the West Indies or the Mediterranean; he is a man of all work, but expert in none — knows a little of many things; but nothing well. He is irregular in his pursuits, "all things by turns," and nothing long, and vain of his ability or information; but is a hardy, frank, good-natured, hospitable, manly fellow, and withal quite as good-looking as his air gives you to understand he thinks himself to be.[21]

---

18 See *A General Description of Nova Scotia* (Halifax, 1823), and Thomas Chandler Haliburton, *An Historical and Statistical Account of Nova Scotia* (Halifax, 1829).

19 McCulloch, *The Mephibosheth Stepsure Letters*, p. 161.

20 Thomas Chandler Haliburton, *The Old Judge, or Life in a Colony* (1849; rpt. Ottawa, 1978), p. 163.

21 *Ibid.*, p. xxi.

The description and the judgment are not unakin to those of Haliburton's earlier literary creation, Sam Slick, who favoured McCulloch's agriculturally-based economy but also saw the need to carry Nova Scotians beyond that base into the Industrial Revolution. Thus, when Sam visits Deacon Flint in the sketch entitled "The Clockmaker," he justifiably admires the trimness of the Deacon's farm and the acreage of his diked land. However, he also sees in the Deacon's water privilege the possibilities of a carding mill, a turning lathe, a shingle machine, and a circular saw. The Deacon's response, "Too old — too old for all those speculations,"[22] neatly sums up the point of Haliburton's satire on his fellow Nova Scotians, for in their unimaginative responses to their natural resources he identifies the reasons why Nova Scotia lags behind America in productivity and wealth. As with McCulloch's *Mephibosheth Stepsure Letters*, the satire is double edged in *The Clockmaker* series, exposing the crassness and boastfulness of the Yankee Sam Slick while revealing the lethargy and lack of confidence of the province's Bluenoses. No sketch better illustrates Sam's technological bent than "Taking off the Factory Ladies" in which Sam visits the Canadian side of Niagara Falls. Impervious to the picturesque qualities of the Falls, he immediately launches into a diatribe on lost industrial opportunities:

> "I guess it is a site," says I, "and it would be a grand spec to git up a joint stock company for factory purposes, for sich another place for mills ain't to be found atween the poles. Oh dear!", said I, "only think of the cardin' mills, fullin' mills, cotton mills, grain mills, sawmills, plaster mills, and gracious knows what sort o' mills might be put up there and never fail for water; any fall you like and any power you want, and yet them goneys the British let all run to waste. It's a dreadful pity, ain't it?"[23]

The scene evokes humour and makes its point because of its exaggeration, but in retrospect it may seem less extravagant when one recalls that its author, Thomas Chandler Haliburton, detected gypsum near the main gates of his home, "Clifton," in Windsor, Nova Scotia, and promptly began to quarry it even though it was only metres away from his front door. "We took a stroll towards the mansion of the veritable Slick, for the purpose of viewing his grounds and appurtenances belonging thereto," noted a traveller in 1841, when suddenly "while journeying in that direction, a load of plaster suddenly broke in upon our view, which appeared to form a bulk, about as large perhaps as a ton of hay.... But our astonishment was soon dispelled — for on approaching a little nearer, we found that the horse and his owner, were

---

22 Thomas Chandler Haliburton, *The Clockmaker* (1836; rpt. Toronto, 1966), p. 9.

23 *Ibid.*, p. 92.

indebted to a railroad, for the convenience with which this mountain of plaster was conducted to its place of deposit, at the wharf."[24] Tea-time at "Clifton" was literally the "machine in the garden" syndrome brought to fruition, an illustration of Haliburton's following the advice of his own literary creation, Sam Slick, when he urged the people to "go ahead."

While the intrusion of the machine into the garden was more literal than allegorical in the case of Thomas Chandler Haliburton, by the late 1830s the yoking of technology and the pastoral had entered Maritime literature, not only because of the practical experience of men like Haliburton, but also through a literary preoccupation with the subject in English and American writing. It is not a pervasive image in Maritime literature, however, and when it does appear in the 1830s and 1840s, it carries connotations of positive rather than negative change. By the 1880s, however, this was to alter as technology, urban growth, consumerism, and scepticism undermined traditional values and the first notes of rural idealization and mythologization began to be struck. Roberts, like Leacock in Ontario, harkened back to a rural and halcyon past. Time for the "Farmer from Cornwallis" in 1789 or for Thomas McCulloch in 1821 or for Thomas Chandler Haliburton in 1835 was money. There were things to do and an energy to be unleashed to do them. Time was stasis by the 1880s when Sir Charles G.D. Roberts caught the Tantramar in memory and vowed to hold it there. Time had wreaked destruction by 1985 when Douglas Lochhead's speaker in *Vigils & Mercies* wanders through the old farm: "The air is heavy with old scents of people, vegetables gone bad, logs rotting in tumbled graves hidden in grass." But lost as the agrarian past of the house seems to be, there is nonetheless life in the voice it awakens. In the "dried up apple" there is a "miracle" of song. "Alone," notes the speaker, "the song becomes mine. The words come from a wizened fruit. Child from a past of orchards. Through a message of blossoms, the kiss of perfume in this old and dying place. Already I forget. It is alive."[25]

24 "Rail Road and Sam Slick — In Windsor," *The Morning News* (Halifax), 27 September 1841. For the "machine in the garden" concept, see Leo Marx, *The Machine in the Garden* (New York, 1964).

25 Lochhead, *Vigils*, pp. 61, 62.

The Song Fishermen:
A Regional Poetry Celebration

"The Twenties," noted Munroe Beattie in *The Literary History of Canada*, were a time of "fresh beginnings," a period when the forces of modernism entered Canadian literature from Europe and the United States and hastened the demise of the romantic Victorian tradition that had so long dominated national writing.[1] Periodicals such as *Poetry: A Magazine of Verse* from Chicago; *transition: an international quarterly for creative experiment* from Paris; *The Canadian Forum*, founded in Toronto in 1920; and *The McGill Fortnightly Review*, established in Montreal in 1925, all helped to broaden both the outlook and the outlets for a new generation of Canadian writers. National poetry, noted Leo Kennedy, "sired by Decorum out of Claptrap," could now begin to be emancipated from the "state of amiable mediocrity" and insipidness in which it had been languishing for so long.[2]

While no student of Canadian literary history can deny the excitement of a period that witnessed the birth of *The Canadian Forum*, the emergence of the Group of Seven, the establishment of *The McGill Fortnightly Review*, the formation of the McGill group of poets, and the growing international experience of writers like Morley Callaghan and John Glassco, it would be remiss for such a student to ignore the central Canadian bias of much that has been said about Canadian writing in the 1920s, or to overlook the emphasis it places on modernism as a yardstick of literary excellence. For this reason, regional romance-writers like Frank Parker Day of Nova Scotia or Margaret Duley of Newfoundland have often been overlooked in analyses of our modern literary development. It is also for this reason that the existence of a small but distinctively romantic group of Nova Scotian poets writing contemporaneously with the McGill group has gone completely unnoticed in *The Literary History of Canada, The Oxford Companion to Canadian Literature,* and other standard discussions of Canadian literary history.

Self-styled "The Song Fishermen," these writers organized lectures and recitals in Nova Scotia, produced illustrated poetry broadsheets, kept in touch with Maritime writers living outside the region, fostered emerging talent (like that of Charles Bruce), published a memorial to Bliss Carman upon his death, and between 1928 and 1930 channelled their energies into the creation of a poetry publication entitled *The Song Fishermen's Song Sheets.* Including such well-known writers as Charles G.D. Roberts, Bliss Carman, James D. Gillis, Andrew Merkel, J.D. Logan, Kenneth Leslie, Charles Bruce, and

---

1   Munro Beattie, "Poetry: 1920-1935," in *The Literary History of Canada* (Toronto, 1976), II, p. 235.

2   *Ibid.*, p. 241.

Robert Norwood, as well as a host of lesser-known versifiers, the Song Fishermen were to represent a Nova Scotian voice in poetry at the very time when rural values and the oral tradition were being eroded by out-migration, a changing economy, and the impact of modern media. As attuned to the developments in modern poetry as were their colleagues in London, Paris, New York or Montreal, the Song Fishermen nonetheless turned to traditional ballads, old sea chanteys, and even Gaelic literary forms in an attempt to evoke what they saw as the essence of Nova Scotia — to convey in the language of the lyric and the ballad their affinity for the sea and their joy in the simple comradeship of the Song Fishermen coterie.

No one who reads the Song Fishermen today can fail to be struck by the sheer exuberance of many of their poems or by the enormous sense of camaraderie permeating the correspondence of the Song Fishermen inner circle. Founded not so much out of a sense of literary purpose as out of a recognition of mutual literary kinship, the Fishermen had their genesis long before the song sheets and broadsheets began to appear in the late 1920s. The key figures from the beginning were always to be the Reverend Dr. Robert Norwood of St. Bartholomews, New York, one of the most prestigious Episcopalian churches in America at the time, and Andrew Merkel of the Canadian Press Office in Halifax. Both men were sons of rural Anglican rectors who had been companions over the years in the Maritimes, Maine and New York. After the death of his father, the young Merkel had even been sent to Hubbards near Halifax to live with the Norwood family for a period of time.[3] A friendship of years and a mutual interest in poetry continued to draw Norwood and Merkel together long after they had embarked on their separate careers, and it was therefore understandable that whenever Norwood was at his summer home in Hubbards, or whenever mutual friends of the two crossed paths, literary and social connections were immediately established. Characteristically, it was Merkel who organized a poetry recital for Norwood in Halifax in 1922, and it was Merkel who in 1923 sent the poetry of Charles Bruce, a student at Mount Allison University, to Maritime writer, Annie Campbell Huestis, in Brooklyn.

Huestis showed this poetry to Robert Norwood in New York,[4] and Norwood subsequently sought out and praised the young poet, Charles Bruce, when he visited Mount Allison on a recital tour on 2 February 1924. After publicly acknowledging the work of Bruce from the stage at Mount Allison, Norwood was to conclude further recitals in his 1924 Maritime tour by

---

3   Andrew Merkel, "Life of Robert Norwood, Outstanding Preacher and Poet, Recalled by Writer," unidentified newspaper clipping, MG 20, vol. 17, 7:3. Public Archives of Nova Scotia (PANS).

4   Robert Norwood to "My dear Mr. Bruce," 22 November 1923, Charles Bruce Papers, Ms. 2, 297, c. 136, Dalhousie University Archives (DUA).

reading not only his own new poem, "The Spinner," but also the verses of his new-found protégé at Mount Allison.[5] A year later when Charles G.D. Roberts, Norwood's former English professor at King's, returned to Canada after living abroad for 30 years, it was only natural that it was to the Merkel household that he gravitated, and that Merkel should invite the young Charles Bruce to Halifax from Sackville to meet Roberts and hear him read at a recital. So pleased was Roberts with his reception in the city that he urged his cousin, Bliss Carman, to favour Halifax with a reading as well,[6] and in the next few years, E.J. Pratt, Wilson MacDonald, Theodore Roberts, and Robert Norwood all complemented the visits of Roberts and Carman by making Halifax a stopping-off place in their literary travels. Their destination invariably included 50 South Park Street, the hospitable home of Andrew Merkel and his wife Tully, "a unique institution," according to Thomas Raddall, that became "the core of the literary life in Halifax for a generation." "For thirty years," recalls Raddall, "the Merkels and their hospitality to writers of every sort made this house famous amongst the fraternity of the pen. Here came Charles and Theodore Roberts, Norwood, Carman, Kenneth Leslie and a host of others who made it their headquarters whenever their footsteps turned homeward to Nova Scotia and the sea."[7]

By 1928 when Charles Bruce had joined the Canadian Press in Halifax under Merkel's tutelage, when Norwood had underwritten the costs of Bruce's first poetry collection, *Wild Apples,*[8] and when Norwood and Roberts had returned to Halifax in September to give a poetry recital together, a strongly unified literary coterie had emerged from the readings, public lectures, and social interconnections that Andrew Merkel had helped to generate and support throughout the 1920s. The result of this was that by October 1928 the group had evolved a dramatic image of themselves as "Fishers of Song," a loosely-connected fellowship of literary fisherfolk who culled from the wind, the sea, and the traditional life style of Nova Scotia the poetic catches that defined their province. Out of the self-romanticization of the Song Fishermen emerged two different publications in the autumn of 1928. One was to be a short-lived series of broadsheets produced under the rubric *Nova Scotia Catches*. The other was to be a more enduring, if less elegantly produced, collection of poems and communications appearing under the title, *The Song Fishermen's Song Sheets*. In the case of the broadsheets, only three seem to have been published, the first one containing

---

5   "Lecture-Recital Was Much Enjoyed," *The Argosy Weekly* (2 February 1924), pp. 2, 5.

6   H. Pearson Gundy, ed., *Letters of Bliss Carman* (Montreal, 1981), pp. 332 and 363; and Andrew Merkel, "Nucleus of Poetry Centre Established in Halifax," unidentified newspaper clipping, Hilda Tyler Collection, MG 1, vol. 925A, PANS.

7   Thomas H. Raddall, *In My Time* (Toronto, 1976), p. 223.

8   Discussion with Harry Bruce, son of Charles Bruce.

the poem "The Bluenose to the Wind" by Andrew Merkel; the second, "On the Road to Maccan" by Kenneth Leslie (an early version of "The Shaunachie Man," his tribute to Robert Norwood); and the third, "Ragwort" by Charles Bruce. Handsomely illustrated and tinted by the artist Donald MacKay who had just returned to Canada after studying with Graham Sutherland in London and at the Académie Colorossie in Paris, the broadsheets also introduced to the public the group's newly established publishing arm, the Abenaki Press. Given this name by Bliss Carman who saw in the ancient tribe of the Abenaki the same affinity to "water and wind and weeds and the human heart"[9] epitomized by the Song Fishermen's poetry, the press proved to be an unprofitable venture in spite of the elegance of its broadsheet productions and the quality of its poetry.

The Song Fishermen were forced, as a result, to fall back on the second of their publishing ventures for a more sustained system of communication. Thus it was that a series of nondescript but serviceable sheets run off on a mimeograph machine in the Halifax office of the Canadian Press became the vehicle of the newly formed Song Fishermen in October 1928. Issued "ever so often"[10] under the editorship of Andrew Merkel and costing a dollar from time to time to cover postage, the publication was to grow from a single sheet of one poem and eleven recipients in the first issue, to twelve sheets and over 60 recipients by the end of its first year. Adding the headnote "Come All Ye" to its masthead in the sixth number (2 December 1928) to signify the oral and balladic root of much of the poetry, the *Song Fishermen's Sheets* also became a vehicle for members' correspondence after the first few issues, affording Bliss Carman, Robert Norwood, Charles G.D. Roberts, and the other non-residents an opportunity to maintain contact with the main Halifax group, as well as to know what was happening to the other members of the coterie scattered from Glace Bay to New York.

From the beginning of the *Song Fishermen's Sheets,* there was a conscious effort on the part of all the participating poets to sustain the marine metaphors and themes that would give focus to an otherwise disparate collection of poetry. The inevitable consequence of this was that a number of the poems seemed to be straining self-consciously for effect rather than to be emerging organically from a central image or idea. The rhetoric of "the catch" (the Song Catches; the "catches are now in the hands of the printer;" "Evelyn Tufts hooks, gaffs, and lands the following")[11] recurred throughout the sheets as a jocular but functional unifying device, and the motif was given further

---

9   *The Song Fishermen's Song Sheet,* 1 (19 October 1928); and "The Song Fishermen" in Charles Bruce to "Dear Mrs. Taylor," 23 August 1966, Charles Bruce Papers, DUA.

10 This phrase appeared in the headnote of each *Song Fishermen's Song Sheet.*

11 See *The Song Fishermen's Song Sheet,* 10 (13 April 1929), p. 3; 2 (25 October 1928), p. 1; and 3 (1 November 1928), p. 1.

play by Eliza Ritchie and Kenneth Leslie several years later when they decided to call prospective poetry collections *Songs of The Maritimes* (1931) and *A Catch of Song* (1933) respectively.[12]

In spite of this self-conscious rhetoric and a large body of verse written just for the sheer fun of it, there emerged in the *Song Fishermen's Sheets* a number of poems that illustrated the talent of the writers, all of whom were initially brought together by friendship but continued to write out of an intense commitment to their craft. Kenneth Leslie's broadsheet poem, "On the Road to Maccan," Martha Ann's concrete poem, "Poor Bob," published in December 1928, Joe Wallace's "The Working Class to Sacco and Vanzetti," in April 1929, Robert Norwood's "Homeward Oars," in May 1929, and Kenneth Leslie's "A Memory of James D. Gillis, Teacher," in June 1929, all illustrate why the *Song Fishermen's Sheets* created excitement amongst critics like Lorne Pierce and John Hanlon Mitchell who were on the mailing list.[13] As well, the group's memorial to Bliss Carman compiled shortly after his death, drew praise for the quality of its poetry and production. Published in pamphlet form as Number 13 of the Song Sheets, it contained Leslie's vigorous tribute, "Go, Lank Rover," echoing the Vagabondia rhythms and youthful spirit that Carman had come to represent to the Song Fishermen.

The success of this publication and the increasing publicity that the *Song Sheets* were receiving convinced Merkel by the summer of 1929 that the sheets had grown beyond their original intention of generating fun and communication and had, instead, reached a calibre of performance warranting a book-length anthology of Song Fishermen poetry. "After the September number comes out," he noted, "we have half intentions of drying out the year's catch, pressing it into drums, and loading it aboard a three-master for ports unknown, perhaps Demerara; in other words, binding some of our songs into a printed book for more permanent and wider distribution."[14] Thus it was that in Number 15 of the *Sheets* Merkel came as close to writing an editorial or stating a rationale for the existence of the group as he was ever to do. What emerged was a restatement of the traditional values and rural lifestyle that he felt to be the informing principle of the Song Fishermen's philosophy and the Song Fishermen's poems:

---

12 Eliza Ritchie's *Songs of the Maritimes* was published by McClelland's of Toronto in 1931. Ken Leslie's *A Catch of Song* was being discussed as a publication of the MacMillan Company in 1933 but did not appear. See a letter from MacMillan's to "Dear Mr. Leslie," 15 December 1933, Kenneth Leslie Papers, MG 1, vol. 2201, no. 10, PANS.

13 J.H.M., "Novascotiana," *The Halifax Chronicle*, 29 December 1929.

14 "Announcement," *The Song Fishermen's Song Sheet*, 15 (29 July 1929), p. 1.

We have been writing for fun, and for our own fun. We are rather isolated down here in Nova Scotia. The material and commercial centre of gravity is distant from us, and has drawn many of our people away. The march of progress goes by us on the other side of the hill. It is a march which leaves little time for playing or singing.

There is always plenty of time here, and it is when time is on your hands that you will sing. Ross Bishop, the clockmaker of Bridgetown, locks his shop, hangs a sign on the door, "Gone Fishing," and goes. You cannot do that in Toronto or New York. Ross has plenty of time on his hands. He plays five or six instruments of music. He studies geology. He is an inventor. He loves to sit quiet in the woods and listen to nothing in particular for no definite length of time. The windows of his soul are open. He does a certain amount of mending clocks, but he does not have to punch them as he did that time he worked up in Waltham.

Let us not get too ambitious. Keep your eyes free from the glare of big cities and big reputations. Keep your mind free from the contemporary illusion which names every new thing a good thing, and turns its back on old things which have been proved in many thousand years of human blood and tears.[15]

For any Maritimer familiar with the forces of change in the region's rural life in the 1920s and 1930s, Merkel's description of small towns seems romanticized and clichéd in *Sheet* Number 15. Yet the Song Fishermen were far too worldly a group not to recognize the influences eroding the idealized Nova Scotia of their poems and of Merkel's editorial. In 1923, Merkel had covered the brutal confrontations between labour and capital in Cape Breton for the Canadian Press, earning the respect of all parties for the fairness of his reporting. His familiarity with Cape Breton had intruded even into the *Song Fishermen's Sheets* when, in February 1929, he responded to Stuart McCawley's contribution of "The Yahie Miners" with his own editorial aside:

We are indebted to Stuart McCawley for The Yahie Miners. He writes it was written about 1884 and is still being sung in Cape Breton. "Yahie," he explains, means "uncouth farmer." He might have added that the ballad deals with a condition that is largely responsible for the difficulties that are encountered in the prosecution of the coal industry in Nova Scotia. Coal mining in Cape Breton is really a seasonal occupation. Before the entry of the Dominion Coal Company the mines were operated for the most part during the summer months when the St.

---

15 *Ibid.*

Lawrence was free from ice and there was ready access to an adequate market. A large proportion of the mine workers were farmers who returned to their homes in the country when navigation closed in the Fall. Since that time efforts to operate the mines continuously have failed because of the limited market offering during the winter months and as a result distress in many of the communities has become a hardy perennial.[16]

Robert Norwood and others amongst the Song Fishermen also had first-hand experience of the economy of the region. Norwood had served in the parishes of Neil's Harbour, Hubbards, and Springhill before moving to urban churches outside the Maritimes, and well knew the precariousness of rural and resource economies. Joe Wallace had already been involved with the Independent Labour Party and the Workers' Party throughout the 1920s, and Kenneth Leslie had begun to demonstrate in his writing that sense of conscience that was to define his later social and political conduct in New York. It was typical of Leslie that when he read Joe Wallace's poem "I brought them forth," he wrote to the *Song Sheets* that Wallace's poem was "an arrow in the throat of despair." For Leslie, Wallace had "spoken the burden of those who suffer when justice bows to power."[17]

Thus, it was probably inevitable that the *Song Fishermen's Sheets* would some day change in tone as the "old things" of Merkel's romanticized Nova Scotia altered. Shades of this had already happened in the *Sheets* with the publication of Wallace's "The Working Class to Sacco and Vanzetti" (13 April 1929) and "The Giant out of a Job" (23 June 1929). Yet neither Merkel nor the other Song Fishermen could have anticipated how quickly the *Song Fishermen's Sheets* were to end. Almost as Merkel wrote of "drying out the year's catch" and "pressing it into drums," the "material and commercial sensibility" he so deplored began to assert itself in a most unexpected form. J.F.B. Livesay, father of the poet Dorothy Livesay and General Manager of the Canadian Press, had, according to Merkel, "many excellent qualities, including a love for poetry, but Livesay decided the Song Sheet, issued not more than once a month and entirely made up to contributions, was taking too much of the time of his Atlantic Superintendent. So he instructed me to dispense with it forthwith."[18]

---

16 For Merkel's response to the Cape Breton situation, see John Mellor, *The Company Store: James Bryson McLachlan and the Cape Breton Coal Miners, 1900-1925* (Toronto, 1983), pp. 205-06; and the *Song Fishermen's Song Sheet*, 8 (14 February 1929), p. 8.

17 "Kenneth Leslie writes," *The Song Fishermen's Song Sheet*, 11 (2 May 1929), p. 1.

18 Andrew Merkel, "Nucleus of Poetry Centre Established in Halifax," unidentified newspaper clipping, Hilda Tyler Collection, MG 1, vol. 925A, no. 14, PANS.

Deprived of a publishing arm because of Livesay's decision, Merkel and the Song Fishermen coterie decided to proceed with a previously discussed Song Fishermen's picnic as a "climax" to their years of conviviality and poeticizing.[19] Thus, they began to organize an elaborately festive marine excursion befitting their nautical metaphor and outrivalling anything concocted by Stephen Leacock in his famous expedition of the Mariposa Belle.[20] Already embarked on a poetry contest in the *Song Sheets* based on a challenge in one of James D. Gillis's paragraphs in *The Cape Breton Giant*,[21] the Song Fishermen arranged for Gillis to judge the anonymous entries, select a winner, and journey down to Halifax from his home at Melrose Hill in Inverness County to be present at the marine excursion and the coronation of a Song Fishermen's Song King. Gillis, a poet, Gaelic singer, and original speaker of the English language, who in the words of Merkel, "just missed being an honest-to-goodness genius,"[22] had been drawn into the Song Fishermen circle in 1928 when some of the coterie had journeyed to Cape Breton to introduce themselves to him. His colourful style in letters to the group had enlivened many a *Song Sheet* correspondence page, and his judgements on the poems in the *Song Fishermen's Sheets* were always original: "Your literature is absolutely pure and safe and will eventually tend to uplift the people more profoundly than forseen, and in agreeable ways."[23]

The two-day celebration, to which Gillis journeyed on 12 and 13 September 1929, began in Halifax on the Thursday evening with a quartet of sea chanteys and a lecture by Robert Norwood on "Poetry and Nova Scotia." The evening's proceedings left an impression on Gillis, who afterwards recalled the event in *The Song Fishermen's Song Sheet*:

> I attended the Song Fishermen's Picnic, whose grace note was a Lecture by Dr. Norwood, of New York City. This Lecture was delivered on the night before the Picnic. The subject was the Modern Poets of N.S. Dr. Norwood is a widely known scholar, theologian, thinker and poet and now refreshed and replenished by a trip to Palestine. I think I am within my rights to say that the Lecture was not often if ever surpassed. He shouldered the most untried and heavy problems, explained the function of mind and its expression in deeds,

19   *Ibid.*

20   Stephen Leacock, "The Sinking of the Mariposa Belle," in *Sunshine Sketches of a Little Town* (Toronto, 1969 [1912]).

21   "All Hands on Deck," *The Song Fishermen's Song Sheet*, 11 (2 May 1929), pp. 8-10.

22   Merkel, "Nucleus of Poetry Centre Established in Halifax."

23   "The following letter has been received from James D. Gillis," *The Song Fishermen's Song Sheet*, 10 (13 April 1929), p. 1.

prose, and poetry — giving special attention to the poets and poetry of Nova Scotia.[24]

The next morning, some 30 Songsters met at the statue of Robbie Burns opposite the Halifax Public Gardens, were piped to a waiting motorcade, boarded a schooner named "The Drama" at Shad Bay (accompanied again by the sound of pipes), and under a sharply snapping Nova Scotia flag, sailed down the coast to East Dover. Here, the "dry-footed"[25] went ashore to visit the school, the church, and the unique rock formation known as Dover Castle while the true fishermen set sail to capture the catch of the day, two large pollack. By two o'clock the entire body had reassembled on shore for fish chowder, and then settled down for the real business of the event — the crowning of Stuart McCawley of Glace Bay as the King of the Song Fishermen. Bob Leslie, whose free verse offended judge James D. Gillis ("If I must read it in seclusion it is wicked or no good."),[26] received a consolation prize of a rhyming dictionary. Stuart McCawley was solemnly crowned by Robert Norwood with a diadem of dulse. James D. Gillis piped and sang in Gaelic, Patricia McGrath gave an exhibition of Highland dancing, and Kenneth Leslie played the violin and sang his own composition, "Bluenose Blues." "The said lyric," Gillis was to note later, "with the music should be generally known. It is most innocent, unobtrusive, almost pathetic. At the same time it plainly shows the best attitude for a young Nova Scotian in the chaos of inevitable opposition if he wants to triumph in the end."[27] The celebration — as did the group — ended in a clasping of hands, a singing of Auld Lang Syne, and a skirl of pipes. Lovers of tradition to the end, the Song Fishermen concluded their poetic lovefest with the same sense of unity and panache that had marked their entire career.

Following the publication of the last *Song Fishermen's Sheet* in the spring of 1930, attempts were made to sustain the output of the group. Theodore Goodridge Roberts had already expressed his admiration for the Song Sheets in the Saint John *Telegraph Journal* of 14 December 1929, and he now offered the Fishermen an outlet in a new journal he was founding. A notice sent to the Song Fishermen participants announced: *"The Song Fishermen's Song Sheet* has found a permanent home, through the courtesy of Theodore Goodridge Roberts, in ACADIE, a semi-monthly magazine which will appear for the first time on April 15, the birthday of Bliss Carman, Canada's best-

---

24. "A Word From J.D. Gillis," *The Song Fishermen's Song Sheet*, 16 (4 April 1930), p. 2.

25 This expression was one used by Charles Bruce to designate those who preferred the land to the sea. It appears in his poem "Biography" in *The Mulgrave Road* (Toronto, 1951), p. 5.

26 "The Entertaining Steersman," *The Song Fishermen's Song Sheet*, 14 (23 June 1929), p., 1.

27 "A Word from J.D. Gillis," p. 2.

loved poet."[28] After representative offerings of the Fishermen had appeared in *Acadie,* however, the idea was dropped. There were some who thought that Robert Norwood might infuse new life into the *Song Sheets,* and in his correspondence with intimate friends like Kenneth Leslie he explored that possibility:

> You are right about the Song Sheet. It must be reborn, and I hope the day will come when I will be in a position to do something definite for it in the way of financial help. And you are quite right about "Acadie." It won't last, but the Song Sheet was a big venture. I learned from Ethel Butler that I am guilty of having killed Cock Robin. She beat me black and blue this summer. I tried to make her see that it was not easy for me that evening to do better than I did, because I, too, was a Song Sheet fisherman, and that what she thought was my levity was really a way of concealing my brooding love for the whole group. I must have blundered, but I certainly put myself into it. Anyway, it is hard for me to function according to program. But that is past, and one day, I hope to prove to the bunch that I have my arms around them all. They are very dear to me.[29]

Even with the best will, however, there were too many forces distracting the group to make it possible for them to reorganize their energies in a coherent way. The Depression of the 1930s was upon people. Ken Leslie was typical of many of the Fishermen in moving away. And within two years, Robert Norwood was dead, struck down prematurely by a coronary thrombosis. His death, like that of Carman, took from the group a spiritual and symbolic centre. The Song Fishermen and their *Song Sheets* therefore slipped into the nirvana of memory, recalled nostalgically by Merkel, Bruce, Leslie and company over the succeeding years, but forgotten by literary historians and by the province once mythologized by their vision of its rural and nautical character.

Only in the subsequent poems of Kenneth Leslie's *By Stubborn Stars* (1938) and Charles Bruce's *The Mulgrave Road* (1951) did something of the Song Fishermen flavour survive the Song Fishermen group. In "Words Are Never Enough," Bruce recalled the "salt in the blood," the "soundless well of knowing,/ That sea, in the flesh and nerves and the puzzling mind/ Of children born to the long grip of its tide"[30] that characterized many of the

28 "Announcement," Kenneth Leslie Papers, MG 1, vol. 2201, no. 7, 1929, PANS.

29 Bob to "Beloved Ken," 6 September 1930, Kenneth Leslie Papers, MG 1, Vol. 2196, Folder 10, no. 7. PANS.

30 Charles Bruce, "Words Are Never Enough" in *The Mulgrave Road* (Toronto, 1951), pp. 26-27.

Song Fishermen's poems. Yet in the end, the inimitable James D. Gillis had the last word on the world "on the other side of the hill" described by Merkel in his editorial of July 1929. In that world, the "march of progress" went on. It was that "progress" that James D. Gillis first noticed when he arrived in Halifax in 1929. "Such discipline of offending travellers has turned multitudes away to auto cars, and pilgrims to more congenial haunts," he noted in the Song Sheets after his visit; "But Halifax is simply a condensed population claiming no prescience or inspiration."[31] In rural life, James D. Gillis and the Song Fishermen found inspiration. In the modern city, they found no "prescience" — nothing to celebrate when "we have been writing for fun, and for our own fun."[32]

---

31 "A Word from J.D. Gillis," p. 2.

32 "Announcement," *The Song Fishermen's Song Sheet*, 15 (29 July 1929), p. 1.

Frank Parker Day's *Rockbound*

On 20 February 1929 an outraged letter appeared in the *Progress-Enterprise* of Lunenburg, Nova Scotia. Signed by the "Offended Citizens of Rockbound," the letter reappeared in untempered form in the *Halifax Herald* on 26 February. Charging that author Frank Parker Day had visited the island of Ironbound off the South Shore of the province "last summer...collecting material" for his "ridiculous" and "notorious" novel *Rockbound,* the letter went on to accuse the writer of portraying "us humble inhabitants of our little island, as ignorant, immoral and superstitious." The image was unjustified, argued the Ironbounders, for "Our Island can boast of three school teachers, and there isn't a child who cannot read and write. We earn our livelihood by honest toil, from Father Neptune and Old Mother Earth." Why, then, "Mr. Day put such a ridiculous book on the market, belittling the inhabitants of his native province, and those who befriended him," was beyond their conception, but they could only suppose that he might "accumulate quite a bit of money" from his enterprise. So too "did Judas Iscariot when he betrayed his Master," they pointed out, and so too did "Castelreigh [sic] who sold his country, and yet in the end cut his throat." Such, they predicted, was "the ending of all ill-gotten gains," and of all those "who betray their countrymen."[1]

The target of the Ironbounders' wrath was at the height of a distinguished career as a scholar, writer, sometime military officer, and president of Union College in Schenectady, New York, at the time that *Rockbound* appeared. Born in the Methodist parsonage in Shubenacadie, Nova Scotia, on 9 May 1881, Frank Parker Day has left vivid impressions of his childhood in "Apology of an Egoist" and *The Autobiography of a Fisherman.* Descended from Irishmen who had immigrated to the Maritimes from Straban, Day early recognized in his clerical father a man more at ease with "trout-fishing, curing horses, making models of boats and schooners and mixing up Asthma Cure" than with preparing sermons and preaching:

> Father was a kind of missionary person who had had some slight training in medicine. He had the obsession that he could cure asthma, a disease prevalent among the fishermen. He was a big powerful, dogmatic man, and his parishioners dared do nothing but get well, after they had swallowed two bottles of his Cure. Certainly the colour, blackish purple, and the smell, rotten eggs, gave testimony to its efficiency. Some of the ingredients were expensive and it was because

---

1   "Letter to the Editor," *Progress-Enterprise* (Lunenburg), 20 February 1929; "New Book Is 'Ridiculous,' Citizens Say," *Halifax Herald*, 26 February 1929.

of the Asthma Cure and a succession of trotting horses, Palmer, Evangeline and Israel Junior, that we endured the life of poverty and often debt. "Christians should be poor," the old man used to say.[2]

Father and son shared a common bond in their love of fishing, and as the family travelled around Nova Scotia from parish to parish the young Day developed the appreciation of outdoor life and knowledge of the province's waterways that were to inform his writing and bring to it an almost spiritual respect for the restorative powers of nature. Moving to Mahone Bay at the age of fourteen and attending school in Lunenburg gave Day an introduction to the South Shore fishery that was to stand him in good stead when he later turned to the writing of *Rockbound*, for it was on the South Shore that he first became interested in "the fleet of vessels that sailed every spring to the Grand Banks and the Labrador to fish for cod."[3] His friendship with Captain Enoch Mason of the "stout schooner *Nova Zembla*" found expression more than 30 years later in the text of *Rockbound* when the captain of the *Sylvia Westner* self-consciously vies to "be home earlier and with a bigger fare than the *Springwood*, the *Nova Zembla,* or the *Sadie Oxner*."[4] It was Captain Mason who also introduced Day to the life of the inshore fisherman by taking the teenager "with him to fish on Green Bank, off our coast." "How happy and miserable I was then!" recalled Day in 1927. "I was seasick most of the time. There was not the slightest convenience, and bobstays are cold and slippery when seas slop around your knees of a brisk morning, but I was learning to be tough and a sailor."[5]

After graduating from Lunenburg and Pictou Academies, Day worked on coastal vessels in the summers and taught in Acacia Villa, Lower Horton, in the winters ("the dreariest of boarding schools ... well-run by a heavy-handed, old fashioned schoolmaster"). In 1900, Day entered Mount Allison University. Here he revelled in the stimulation of sports, friendships, and academic studies, remembering years later that "I used to feel that my brain was growing, as I sat at my little deal table and tried to solve in my mind some complicated syllogism in the back of Jevon's Logic."[6] The result of the Mount Allison years was not only an abiding affection for his *alma mater* and its strong sense of fellowship but also a Rhodes Scholarship to Oxford in 1905. Entering Christ Church as a candidate in literature, Day approached this experience with the same thirst for life that seemed characteristic of all

---

2   "Apology of an Egoist," B(ib), p. 14, Frank Parker Day Papers, typescript, Dalhousie University Archives (DUA).

3   Day, *The Autobiography of a Fisherman* (Garden City, New York, 1927), p. 45.

4   Day, *Rockbound* (Garden City, 1928), p. 192.

5   Day, *Autobiography of a Fisherman*, p. 46.

6   *Ibid.*, pp. 67, 79.

his endeavours. "Oxford," he was to write later, "is a glorious place to loaf and think and learn slowly...I had a wonderful time there; servants, luxury, theatres, beautiful buildings, pictures, music, burst upon me all at once."[7] In the next two years, he rowed for Christ Church, won the Oxford-Cambridge heavyweight boxing championship, became a lieutenant in the King's Colonials Light Horse, and graduated with honours in English after work with Walter Raleigh, then completing his "English Men of Letters" book on Shakespeare. The year 1907-08 was spent at Berlin University as an assistant to Professor Alois Brandl, but Day returned to Oxford the following year to work on an M.A. and to take up a post as an instructor in English at Bristol University. By the fall of 1909 he was back in Canada as a member of the English Department at the University of New Brunswick. In 1910 he married Yarmouth-born artist and Mount Allison graduate Mabel Killam, who later provided the cover design for his novel, *River of Strangers*. The outbreak of war interrupted an appointment to the English Department at the Carnegie Institute of Technology in Pittsburgh, and during the next five years Day served with the 85th Canadian Infantry Battalion, raised and commanded the 185th Cape Breton Highlanders, and in France commanded the 25th Battalion of the 5th Brigade, Second Division. Promoted a colonel on the field of battle at Amiens, he later integrated some of his war experiences into the *Roses of Mercatel*, "The Iroquois," *The Autobiography of a Fisherman*, and the unpublished "Apology of an Egoist."[8] Described by his son as an illustration of the well-known adage "Old soldiers never die but simply fade away,"[9] Day was to call upon his military background again in the Second World War when he organized a COTC Command Office at Mount Allison, helped plan a POW camp in New Brunswick, and wrote a series of books on basic English for Canadian servicemen.

After returning to North America in 1919, Day re-entered academic life, becoming director of the Division of General Studies at the Carnegie Institute (1919-26), professor of English at Swarthmore College (1926-28), and eventually president of Union College, Schenectady (1928-33). In 1927 Mount Allison awarded him an honorary Doctor of Laws degree and in 1929 New York University followed suit by making him a Doctor of Literature. In spite of his busy academic schedule Day retained an ongoing relationship with his native Nova Scotia throughout this period, often making summer

7   Biographical and Autobiographical Notes, Day Papers, typescript, B2, pp. 1-2, DUA.

8   *Roses of Mercatel*, with words by Frank P. Day and music by J. Vick O'Brien, was presented by the Carnegie Institute of Technology School of Music in Pittsburgh on 8 February 1920. The text and program can be found in *ibid.*, J82 and J86. "The Iroquois" was published in *The Forum*, LXXIV, 5 (November 1925), pp. 752-64.

9   Donald Day to Miss Lewis, 22 November 1972, Day Papers, Biographical and Autobiographical Notes, B2, p. 3, DUA.

visits or fishing expeditions to the province. By the time *Rockbound* appeared in 1928, it was clear that Nova Scotia was central to his literary imagination. "An Epic of Marble Mountain" (1923) and *River of Strangers* (1926) both drew on the Cape Breton background that Day had come to know so well in his wartime training and experience, and *The Autobiography of a Fisherman* (1927) integrated Day's Nova Scotian experiences with his exploration of man's place in the natural and social scheme of things:

> As for me, I endure the city in winter in order that I may live through three long summer months. In the city, I write endless letters in my office, I am busy over executive work, I rush about day and night getting only half enough sleep, my mind full of ambitious and often angry thoughts. But in summer, all is different: in a country almost untouched by man, I get up fresh and clear eyed to watch the sun rise out of the forest and chase the mist wraiths from the lake, I take my canoe and paddle over to the still-water for trout, I swim in the cool clean water, I gather pond lilies and berries in season, I cut wood or hoe my garden or drive back the forest of alders that is forever encroaching. I explore some new part of the forest, boil my kettle by some singing brook, and lie in the sun for hours. A lazy life, you say, yet life, after all, with one's head full of sweet dreams and fancies. At night, I build up a log fire, for it is always a little chilly in the evenings, and by the light of a shaded oil lamp settle down in my armchair with a book I love.[10]

Moments of relaxation like these were few for Day. As he wrote Nella Broddy of Doubleday, Page & Company in 1923, he could find little time in his busy academic schedule for writing the stories and novels so important to him.[11] None the less, surviving notes, letters, and drafts all indicate that he was working on *Rockbound* in the mid-1920s even as his first novel, *River of Strangers,* was still with the publishers. Day had vivid memories of the rugged coast of Nova Scotia's South Shore from his two years of living there as a youth, and his periods of fishing with Captain Enoch Mason had provided him with an introduction to the rigours of a fisherman's life. These first-hand experiences clearly played a part in the shape and design of *Rockbound* as Day began to work on the novel, and manuscript stories like "The Footless Nigger" and "The Ghost-Catcher" indicate his experimentation with South Shore folk tales that might be incorporated into the text of the narrative.[12] However the key element in filling in the background of

---

10 *Autobiography of a Fisherman*, pp. 73-74.

11 Day to Miss Nella Broddy, 12 December 1923, Day Papers, C60, DUA.

12 "The Footless Nigger," Ts.ss.G14 and "The Ghostcatcher," G15, *ibid.*

Rockbound, Barren Island, and the Outposts in the novel lay in Day's visit to Ironbound, Pearl Island, and the Tancooks in the summer of 1926. Here he began to scribble descriptive notes, names of people, ghost stories, island gossip, and interesting expressions ("to rutch up") into a working journal and text begun on 30 July 1926 on Ironbound. The ballad sung by Gershom in the fish house scene in the novel is copied into the notes under the title "How Israel's Prayer Was Answered." A visit to the Smith's Cove cemetery to check the accuracy of local names introduced him to "Gershom" and eventually led to his changing the name of the "blonde Viking" from "Mather" in one working draft to Gershom in the final version. He also made lists of books that light keepers had read on Pearl (Barren) Island, researched the bird life existing in the offshore islands, and consulted Mather Byles DesBrisay's *History of Lunenburg County* (1870) for background information.[13]

Nowhere is Day's on-the-spot integration of South Shore life into the novel better illustrated, however, than in his response to the tragic events of 7-9 August 1926, when a Caribbean storm swept up the Atlantic and battered schooners of the Lunenburg fleet fishing off the coast of Sable Island. Headlines and articles from the *Halifax Herald,* the *Halifax Morning Chronicle,* and the *Yarmouth Telegram* from 11-19 August were clipped out and glued into Day's draft of "The Summer Storm" in *Rockbound* as the tragic fate of the *Sylvia Mosher* and the *Sadie Knickle* unfolded in the newspapers.[14] Day's *Sylvia Westner* in the novel is a fictional ship, but her captain, crew, and destiny find close parallel to those of the *Sylvia Mosher* described in the *Herald* and the *Morning Chronicle*. Like the *Sylvia Mosher's* Captain John D. Mosher, memorialized by the newspaper as "one of the youngest skippers in the Lunenburg fleet and high-liner for the last three years," Day's Captain Johnny Westner is the "smartest young skipper on all the coast" with a schooner that "had been for three seasons high-line of all the Liscomb fleet."[15] The crew, as one newspaper noted, had been carefully selected, for "the Sylvia Mosher being a hand liner, took the pick of the young men, the brightest, ablest, finest men of the community."[16] In the novel, Uriah takes great pride in his Rockbounders being asked to serve on the *Sylvia Westner*, for "Johnny Westner, smartest young skipper on all the coast, picked only the most skilled hand-liners and ablest men for his

---

13   Manuscript Rockbound (Ironbound), E4C (i) and (ii), pp. 99-100, 161, 102-03, 210-14, 257-58, *ibid.*

14   *Ibid.,* pp. 176-81, 215-25.

15   See "Lunenburg Schooner 'Sylvia Mosher' Total Loss on Sable Island Bar: No Trace of Fishing Captain and Crew," *Halifax Herald,* 11 August 1926, and *Rockbound,* p. 174.

16   "Sea is Strewn With Wreckage, But There is No Sign Of Life," *Morning Chronicle* (Halifax), 13 August 1926.

crews."[17] In at least one case, Day made no distinction between a factual and a fictional crew member, for Caleb Baker of the LaHave Islands appears in the newspaper as a missing member of the *Sylvia Mosher* complement and in the novel as a helmsman from the La Tuque Islands.[18] The most striking example of the integration of documentary into fiction, however, lies in the description of the *Sylvia Mosher/Sylvia Westner* sinking off Sable Island. The *Mosher* was at anchor some 30 miles south of Sable when the storm broke, according to the *Halifax Herald*, and from the evidence it seems that Captain Mosher decided to run with light canvas before the wind and head toward the western end of the island:

> It would only require a flying jib sail to send the craft bowling along at a fast rate before such a wind. The island was rapidly approaching. West Light was showing up on the port bow. Stygian blackness and only the flashing hope of the sailors' friend as a guide. Hauling off before such a wind might send her into the vortex of raging breakers ahead, broadside on to certain destruction. She had crossed this western bar before. There were numerous channels. It was high water. Anyway to turn back now was impossible. Through the hissing foam-lashed breakers she must go — and through the other side to safety and shelter in the lee of the island on the northern side. But the doomed vessel did not win through.
>
> With the hurricane driving her sheer hull through the spumedrift and tempest-lashed shallow water over the bar at a speed calculated to be anything between twelve to sixteen knots, she grounded on a shoal, her whole bottom was ripped asunder in one fell sweep and she turned over and over, her masts wrenched completely from their holdings in the keelson and everything movable, living and inanimate gone in one catastrophic crash that could have taken but moments to happen.[19]

The vividness of the *Halifax Herald* account obviously fuelled Day's imagination as he plotted the last minutes of the *Sylvia Westner's* voyage. In the novel, Captain Johnny decides that "the only chance was to drive straight on before the gale." Knowing that when "the tide was at the top of the flood, there were deep channels through the sand," he tries to run the *Sylvia Westner* over the western bar of Sable Island:

---

17 *Rockbound*, p. 174.

18 "Lunenburg Schooner," *Herald*, and *Rockbound*, p. 193.

19 "'Sylvia Mosher' is Battered Derelict," *Herald*, 19 August 1926.

Wind furies shrieked, stays and halliards groaned with the straining spars, piled dories tugged at their lashings, a water butt broke loose and went booming along the deck to crash into the forecastle hatch. A mountain of white water gathered behind the *Sylvia Westner,* rose with slow, malicious dignity, and crashed down upon her poop....

At that moment the *Sylvia Westner* struck; Hand-line Johnny had no luck that night. All was over in the twinkling of an eye. The vessel, deep-laden, was travelling at the rate of twenty knots, and a tooth of black bottom rock whipped bottom and keelson from her as cleanly as a boy with a sharp jackknife slits a shaving from a pine stick. Two thousand quintals of split fish and the unwetted salt dropped down upon the yellow sands; out came the spars with a rending crash, and deck and upper hull turned over. Within ten seconds of her striking, every man of the crew was in the sea.[20]

The malignancy of the storm, the reference to the Sable Island light, the hope of channels through the bar, the moment when rock lacerates the hull, and the image of men and fish tossed to the sand and the sea all link Day's imaginative depiction of the sinking to the *Halifax Herald's* reconstruction of actual events. Episodes like this one prompted Archibald MacMechan to write Day on 27 October 1928 to congratulate him on "bringing realism into Canadian fiction." "You have got rid of convention and polite periphrasis," noted the Dalhousie professor and critic. "You have given us life, in the raw actuality."[21] MacMechan's claim may have been somewhat dramatic, but the working manuscripts of *Rockbound* and the surviving letters and notes surrounding the composition of the novel leave no doubt of Day's search for authenticity. A sketch of Pearl Island, the model for Barren Island in the novel, reveals the location of buildings, fishing grounds, net, trawl and even a "groaner" or bellows buoy to the south of the island. The detail on a mock-up of Ironbound (Rockbound) includes trees, pastures, houses, and the place where a "whale ran ashore in the olden days." And a working map of Mahone Bay includes actual place names of mainland and island locations appearing in the novel with Day's fictional adaptation of those names. Thus, Ironbound becomes Rockbound, Big Tancook becomes Big Outpost, Blandford is Sandford, Chester is Minden, and Lunenburg becomes Liscomb. Sacrifice Island, Big Duck, Little Duck, and the Bull remain unchanged in the transition from geographical fact to fiction. Even specific buildings seem to be thoroughly researched by Day as he develops a visual sense in his novel. A sketch of the lighthouse on Pearl Island reveals it to be the inspiration of

20   *Rockbound*, pp. 195-96.
21   Archibald MacMechan to Day, 27 October 1928, Day Papers, C277, DUA

Gershom's lighthouse on Barren Island in the novel. Integrated into a draft text of *Rockbound,* the sketch reveals everything from the placement of guy ropes on the outside of the structure to the location of a bookcase in the interior. That Day was actually working with a first-hand knowledge of the building emerges in his manuscript notes, for number 19 on his sketch is marked, "Upper room where Mather & I drank rum & talked till 1:30 after the women slept," and number "3 = 6" includes the note, "Table where I wrote on the sly pretending I was preparing Shakespeare lecture."[22]

It was Day's discretion in gathering realistic detail for his novel that no doubt escalated the tension between the Ironbounders and Day after the publication of *Rockbound* and further precipitated the letter to the Lunenburg *Progress-Enterprise* from the "Offended Citizens of Rockbound." Certainly, surviving correspondence from local residents after the summer of 1926 does not give any indication that people were aware of Day's research intent when he visited the islands. Writing to Day on 22 September 1926, one lighthousekeeper thanked him for sending a copy of H. G. Wells's *The Outline of History,* noted that he had caught "a 200 lb. Halibut" the "next day after you left," and observed that "It is lovely out here at this time of year cool days and lots of sport — good rum and brandy & wine. I was ashore for a week and had a change." Similarly, three letters from an islander in the Blandford post office district are filled with news of people Day knew, acknowledgments for seeds that he had sent after visiting, and a request that Day purchase a "10 gage hammer gun" on his behalf "when you come down" next. In a letter dated 31 January 1927, the correspondent remarked: "I have heard you have written a book and we would all like very much to read it, would you tell me where to buy it. I would be very much interested in new book of eny kind and especially the one you wrote."[23] Given the fact that Day was still negotiating with Doubleday, Page & Company for the publication of *Rockbound* as late as the following summer, it seems likely that the book being discussed is either *River of Strangers* or *The Autobiography of a Fisherman.* However, there is no question that it is *Rockbound* to which a former islander referred when he wrote to Day on 2 May 1929, two months after the Ironbound letter in the *Progress-Enterprise.* Noting that he had recently moved to the mainland, he went on to say: "My object in writing is to see if you can secure for me a copy of your book (Rockbound). I've been trying to get hold of it ever since it came on the market but seemingly cannot. They have it at Ironbound but will not send it no doubt they blame me altho I am not sure for spilling myself to you at any rate they are wild about it."

In responding on 18 May 1929, Day apologized for not forwarding a copy of *Rockbound* but explained that he had none available. "I am very sorry that

22 *Ibid.,* E4C (i), p. 89e; E4C (ii), n.p.; E4J; E4C, p. 96.

23 *Ibid.,* C329, to Day, 22 September 1926; C455, to Day, 31 January 1927.

the people of Ironbound have been in any way offended," he said, "as the story is not intended to be about them nor did I get any information whatsoever from you. The story refers to a time long ago not to present-day conditions and I learned many of the stories when I was a little boy before I had ever heard of Ironbound."[24] In spite of Day's denials, feelings against him did not die easily on the islands, as author Thomas H. Raddall pointed out in his 1976 autobiography *In My Time*. Engaged by *Maclean's Magazine* in 1946 to do an article on Tancook Island, Raddall chatted to a local doctor in Chester as he prepared to board the ferry to Tancook:

> He warned me not to reveal myself as a writer. In the mid-1920s a literary professor named Frank Parker Day had spent two or three summers on Tancook's small neighbour, Ironbound Island, whose people are all close blood relations of the Tancookers. In 1928 he published a pseudo-novel called *Rockbound*, portraying the Ironbounders as a backward folk, the result of generations of intermarriage, speaking English with a thick Old German accent, and lusty in their quarrels and amours. According to the doctor, Day never returned to Ironbound. The Tancookers and Ironbounders would have hanged him if he did.[25]

As late as 1980 there were still elderly residents of the South Shore who spoke disparagingly of Day's novel and of the impression of Ironbounders and Tancookers that it had created.[26]

Ironically, Day's early draft of *Rockbound* contained little of the material that was to offend Ironbound residents in 1929. A short typescript version found in Day's papers at the Dalhousie University Archives has a cast of islanders named Harris, Uriah, and Mary Mader. There is no Gershom Born figure in this story, possibly the one submitted to Doubleday, Page & Company in 1925 or early 1926 to test the publisher's interest.[27] In it, a New

---

24   *Ibid.*, C240, to Day, 2 May 1929; from Day, 18 May 1929.

25   Raddall, *In My Time: A Memoir* (Toronto, 1976), pp. 255-56.

26   Over the years a number of Nova Scotians have told me of the unfavourable response of South Shore residents to *Rockbound* when it appeared in 1928. Around 1980 I sat next to an elderly Lunenburg woman at the annual banquet of the Royal Nova Scotia Historical Society in Halifax. She expressed great dismay when she learned that I was teaching *Rockbound* to my students at Mount Allison University. Her family had come from Ironbound and Big Tancook and the novel was still an anathema to her.

27   Day to Nella Broddy Henney, 28 January 1926, Day Papers, C60. In this, Day says: "I am glad you think there is a book in "Ironbound" and I am going to work on that this summer." Writing to Day on 31 January 1927 Allan Davis, a Pittsburgh lawyer, refers to "the first Iron Bound sketch that you read at the Authors' Club a couple of years ago." (C100) In all

York artist named Antriquet comes to the island, wins Mary from Harris, and goes off to New York with her at the end. References to daily life and to the rugged individualism of the islanders do provide some sense of local colour in this working text, but there is none of the rich, regional dialect that was to bring verbal vitality to *Rockbound*. When Uriah and the Young Harris (later David) meet for the first time on Ironbound in the draft, their conversation is in conventional English:

> At eighteen when he heard that his great great uncle Uriah, the rich king of Ironbound wanted a man, he rowed out in a dory and applied for the job.
> "We work here on Ironbound," said the old man.
> "I know how to work."
> "Know how to work and from Tancook," said Uriah scornfully. "We've half a day's work done here before Tancookers begin to rub their eyes."
> "Try me," replied the boy.
> "Where's your gear and clothes?"
> "I got all my gear and clothes with me," said Harris, grinning down at his ragged trousers. "I own yon dory, I salvaged from the sea and beat the man who tried to take her from me." Uriah's eyes showed a glint of interest.[28]

Between the writing of this draft version entitled "Ironbound" and the submission of the work to Doubleday, Page & Company in the spring of 1927, Day seems to have revised the novel to capture the distinctive flavour of the "Lunenburg Dutch" spoken along the South Shore of the province. A form of English that evolved amongst the descendants of the German settlers who immigrated to the area in the eighteenth century, Lunenburg Dutch retains some of the syntactical and phonological features of German speech. The result, as Kirsten Stevens has pointed out, is that Uriah will say "I'se'll let him go wid as a favour" instead of "I will let him go with you as a favour." "Ain't" or "ain't it" often end statements seeking confirmation, "v" becomes "w" in words like "wery" and "wisit," and consonants like "d" and "t" become substitutes for the "th" sound ("He had dat wery audacious Sanford Ghos'"). It is this distinctive speech pattern that Mary Dauphiny tries to correct when she begins to teach Fanny, David, and the children in the new school on Rockbound. "You and Fanny have got to stop saying 'wid' and 'dat,'" she tells David, as she "put her tongue between her closed teeth and

likelihood, the typescript of "Ironbound" is the one read at the Authors' Club and possibly shown to Doubleday.

28 *Ibid.*, Ts.G27.

showed them how to say 'th'...Then David and Fanny each had to say 'that' and 'with' fifty times with much spluttering, spitting, and suppressed laughter...."[29]

In practical terms, Mary's attempts to homogenize Rockbound speech are part of a process of social change on the island that also sees engines replacing oxen at the launch and Casper's going out west on a harvest excursion. In literary terms, however, Mary's educated speech lacks the uniqueness of idiom and syntax found in the oral tradition. Day's self-conscious effort to make a record of expressions, pronunciations, and names when he visited the islands in the summer of 1926 and his integration of that research into scenes like the opening Uriah-David confrontation reveal the painstaking diligence with which he revised the manuscript to make it as dramatic and authentic as possible. As Stevens has noted, instead of the "we work here on Ironbound" structures of the early draft, the reader of the final version has a sense of the rugged isolation that has preserved the originality of both character and speech on the island:

> "An' what might ye be wantin'?" said the old man, the king of Rockbound.
> "I wants fur to be yur sharesman," answered David.
> "Us works here on Rockbound."
> "I knows how to work."
> "Knows how to work an' brung up on de Outposts!" jeered Uriah. "Us has half a day's work done 'fore de Outposters rub de sleep out o' dere eyes, ain't it!"
> "I knows how to work," repeated the boy stubbornly.
> "Where's yur gear an' clothes at?"
> "I'se got all my gear an clothes on me," said David grinning down at his buttonless shirt, ragged trousers and bare horny feet, "but I owns yon dory: I salvaged her from de sea an' beat de man what tried to steal her from me."
> Uriah's eyes showed a glint of interest.[30]

By the time that Day submitted the novel to Doubleday, Page & Company in the spring of 1927, it had gone through a number of drafts and had been

---

29 *Rockbound*, pp. 120, 163; Kirsten Allegra Stevens, "Speech in Selected Works of Three Maritime Authors," B.A. thesis, Mount Allison University, 1981, pp. 35-36, also 40-41. Stevens quotes H. Rex Wilson, "Lunenburg Dutch: Fact and Folklore" in J.K. Chambers, ed., *Canadian English: Origins and Structures* (Toronto, 1975).

30 *Rockbound*, pp. 4-5.

read by at least two discerning friends.[31] Referred to at various points in Doubleday's correspondence as "The Devil's in the Sea," "The Devil's Island," and "The Islanders," the novel was initially returned to Day on 1 June 1927 with the suggestion that he tighten the point of view. The scene with the sinking of the *Sylvia Westner* was praised by the editors, although Day was encouraged to expand or delete the confrontation between Gershom and the devil.[32] In letters of 2 March and 15 March 1928, Doubleday, Doran & Company enthusiastically accepted Day's re-submitted manuscript, offering him a royalty of "10% until our plant account is paid, 12 1/2% on the next 2500, and 15% thereafter."[33] There were suggestions that Day might make the sinking of the *Sylvia Westner* even more vivid and that he might reconsider his use of Shakespeare's *The Tempest* in the text, but publication was none the less assured. A follow-up letter from Beecher Stowe of Doubleday on 30 April 1928 explained somewhat apologetically that the publisher had "taken the liberty of slightly modifying certain words and phrases in your manuscript which it seemed to us might give unnecessary offense to a considerable number of readers.... For example, where you say 'God Damn' I have cut out the 'God'." Correspondence about editorial changes and the title continued until the end of June when publisher and author both decided to change the name to *Rockbound* even though the dies for another title had already been cast and the book was in galleys.[34]

By the late fall of 1928, *Rockbound* was being reviewed in a number of American newspapers. Responses were favourable if misguided, often placing the novel on the Grand Banks or identifying Day as a Newfoundlander who returned to his native area "every summer to fish and sail." Commentators frequently confused Day's nationality as much as they did his geography, describing him as a Rhodes scholar from the United States, or, in the words of the Dallas *Times-Herald,* "an Englishman who has spent much of his scholastic life in London, Berlin and Heidelberg" but "likes

---

31 Friends wrote to Day on 31 January (C100) and 10 April 1927 (C252) about the working versions of *Rockbound*. Allan Davis had obviously seen a version of the novel written between the "Ironbound" typescript (which may have been the draft he had heard Day read at the Author's Club in Pittsburgh a couple of years before) and the final one; he advised Day to focus the book on one central character more than he had done and to eliminate an artist theme that he had included. The other friend had been reading a version of the novel not unlike the published one, and advised Day to tighten the point of view in the novel. Both urged Day to develop the psychology of the female character (Polly/ Mary) in greater depth. Both felt he was working with epic material and expressed their admiration for what he was writing.

32 Nella B. Henney to Day, 1 June 1927, *ibid.*, C60.

33 Nella B. Henney to Day, 2 and 15 March 1928, *ibid.* Day agreed to the financial arrangements on 20 April 1928 (M3).

34 Beecher Stowe to Day, 30 April, 8 May and 26 June 1928, *ibid.*, C401.

best to live and work in America and feels he would not be content anywhere else." The *New York Herald-Tribune* of 9 December confirmed the Ironbounders' worst fears by noting that "A woman with the morals of a mink is pictured as the dear chum of the school teacher" and that "It is true that there are people of rabbit morals living on the outer islands of Maine and Canada...."[35]

In his native Canada, Day fared somewhat better in the accuracy accorded both his book and his background, but his distance from literary circles in Toronto militated against his receiving much national attention. In a review in *Saturday Night* entitled "Heroic Mould," author Raymond Knister set his discussion of *Rockbound* in the context of Day's previous fiction, praising the story "An Epic of Marble Mountain" published in *Harper's Magazine* in September 1923 and describing the novel *River of Strangers* as "distinctly a cut above average." The mores and the conversation of the Rockbounders struck Knister as being "very crude," but he praised Day for being an author who "does not blink them." "There is nothing here of the evangelical or the idyllic," he noted. "Rather does the story, its swift telling, and the full-lunged men and women call for the word epic. Epic breadth of material and of language."[36]

The mythic or epic proportions of the tale also caught the attention of two other Canadian reviewers. Detecting an almost naturalistic relationship between "the crass superstition, the low moral standards.... The ignorance and quarrelsomeness" of Day's characters and the restrictedness and harshness of their living conditions, Eliza Ritchie of the *Dalhousie Review* none the less praised the "unfailing courage and intense laboriousness" of "the Atlantic fishermen's heritage" depicted in the novel. A Wellesley College professor who had returned to her native Nova Scotia, Ritchie was not uncritical of the "commonplace" love interest and ending of the book. On the whole, however, she found "With no sentimentality, and but little romance, there is an almost epic strength and largeness in the atmosphere of the story."[37]

The other major Canadian review also responded to the "stark realism" and epic sweep of the tale, introducing into its text such phrases as "turbulent epic," "Viking pioneers," "Norse hero," and "supremacy of man...working with Destiny." Written by J.D. Robbins of the *Canadian Forum*, it countered Eliza Ritchie's implications of naturalism in the novel by declaring that "Back of Rockbound...is the sense of the supremacy of man again, working with Destiny if you will, but achieving by means of an indomitable will

---

35 *Ibid.*, Book Reviews, M2, Sacramento *Bee*, 26 November 1926, and Dallas *Times-Herald*, 25 November 1928; Wilbert Snow, "A Professor's Novel," *New York Herald-Tribune*, 9 December 1928, section XI, 21.

36 Raymond Knister, "Heroic Mould," *Saturday Night* (December 1928).

37 E.R., "New Books," *Dalhousie Review*, IX, 1 (April 1929), p. 129.

which can send even Destiny to its purpose."[38] Robbins was particularly drawn to the fish-shed scene during the herring run when "on an unimaginably fatiguing Saturday night" the "blood and filth and sweat are cleansed away from the reader's mind by the old hymn of Fanny the fish-girl." It was this realism that Mazo de la Roche praised when she noted the "fine simplicity" of *Rockbound's* "hard bitten fishermen."[39] The novel was "without sugar and without rose-pink," added Archibald MacMechan in a letter to literary historian Ray Palmer Baker: "He [Day] has caught the life of Lunenburg. Absolutely. Enter Realism on the amateur stage of Canadian fiction."[40]

MacMechan's reference to the "amateur stage of Canadian fiction" reflects his consciousness of literary change in the 1920s. James Joyce had published *Ulysses* in 1922. Gertrude Stein had uncategorically proclaimed her generation lost. And there was an explosion of literary and publishing energy throughout North America and Europe that saw Day's titles competing in bookstores with those of F. Scott Fitzgerald, D.H. Lawrence, Ernest Hemingway, and Sinclair Lewis. In Canada the Group of Seven, the *Canadian Forum,* and the McGill Group were challenging old shibboleths, while in the United States a decade of rapid social development had found literary expression in a new emphasis on form and irony.

For Day, like many others, this period was one of enormous cultural shifts. Raised in a rural Nova Scotian environment that saw the novel "as something depraved if not essentially wicked," Day harkened back to values, virtues, and codes that made him a forceful leader among his peers but a reluctant catalyst for literary change. Thus, his ideal in fiction still lay with the great classics of Richardson, Eliot, Meredith, Dickens, and the other novelists of character. The two significant developments in the history of the genre, as Day argued them, were a growing democratization of character in the eighteenth and nineteenth centuries and a shift in emphasis from outward life to inward life. "We do insist on knowing about hero and heroine," he noted as he addressed his audiences of the 1920s in a lecture entitled "Some Aspects of Modern Fiction": "what they think and feel; we insist on knowing their ideas — if they have any — we want to get their point of view in regard to the world and life. Thus the psychological novel has arisen in the hands of great artists like Eliot and Meredith, and these artists have laid bare to us the souls of their characters. The psychological treatment of characters has in fact gone over to all novelists and influenced them."[41]

---

38   J.D. Robbins, "Viking Pioneers," *Canadian Forum,* IX, 103 (April 1929), p. 245.

39   A. Page Cooper to Day, 22 November 1928, Day Papers, C87.

40   Archibald MacMechan to Ray Palmer Baker, *ibid.,* C277.

41   "Some Aspects of Modern Fiction," pp. 2, 7, Essay, K10, *ibid.*

In spite of Day's statements on the importance of interiority in the novel and his own attempts to develop that emphasis in *John Paul's Rock* in 1932, he remained comparatively untouched by the modernist tendency to make ethical considerations secondary to those of form, language, and style. By contrast, the novel "that lifts one from the dull grey world in which we live, a grey world full of incompatibility, divorce and the thousand ills that flesh is heir to," was the novel that Day admired. "Surely the function of the artist is not to depict life photographically," he argued, "but to help us to interpret the beauty of life as it may be, to present to us romance, adventure, idealism, and to reveal the nobility lying latent in every human breast."[42]

Romance, adventure, idealism, and latent nobility underlie David Jung's struggle in *Rockbound* and ensure that after a period of testing he can forego a "turfy path" for "a way of gold, full of flowers, not of this earth, but like to those with which medieval painters adorned their foregrounds."[43] The Garden of Eden that David creates out of Barren Island, the fable-like Story of the King, the Empress, the young trojan, and the Blond Giant, and the implacable confrontation of the devil, Gershom, and Uriah, all bring an element of romance to the work that places it in a continuum of story-telling from the Old Testament to the present. Day's classical allusions and literary references further enhance the universality of the novel, linking the straightforward heroism of the Rockbounders to a well of human emotion and experience. The timeless story patterns, Chaucerian headnotes, and analogies to Shakespeare's *The Tempest* were not enough to convince irate Ironbounders that Day intended the general rather than the specific, however. Nor is there any question that the appeal of the novel lies in the detail of its island life. Day-to-day rhythms linked to the sea and the weather, patterns of domestic routine and gossip, intricacies of land feuding, lighthouse-tending, the herring run, and the islanders' pragmatic mingling of Old Testament theology and superstition all give *Rockbound* a distinctive texture of local colour. Moreover, more than any other English-Canadian novel of its period, *Rockbound* conveys a sense of the folk-life of its constituency, particularly in its integration of tale-telling, balladry, and ghost stories into the pattern of the narration. Uriah understands his people well when at the height of the herring scene he can offset their weariness by prevailing on Gershom to "Speak us a piece...speak us one ye made yur own self."[44] The resulting ballad draws on irony, mock religious rhetoric,[45] and the appeal of hypocrisy, greed, and cuckoldry as enduring themes. Uriah pretends to be shocked, but he is as

---

42 "Modern Novelists: John Masefield as Representative of that Group," p. 4. Essays, K6, *ibid*.

43 *Rockbound*, p. 292.

44 *Rockbound*, p. 59.

45 Debra A. Surette, "Folklore in *Rockbound* and *John Paul's Rock*," B.A. thesis, Mount Allison University, 1981, pp. 18-19.

taken as are his followers with the audaciousness of Gershom's irreverence. Throughout the novel, Rockbounders take no chance with heaven, but they also exhibit an enduring belief in fate, destiny, and the supernatural as being potentially as powerful as their Old Testament God. Thus, it is perfectly natural that the devil should appear to Gershom in the guise of a fisherman, for whether it be the philosophical David, the romantic Gershom, or the grasping Uriah, all Rockbounders believe that "the devil" is "in the sea."[46] The "supernatural in Nova Scotia is not a subject talked about for the sole purpose of entertainment," Helen Creighton has pointed out in *Bluenose Ghosts,* "but for many of us," she adds, "it is part of our way of life."[47] Day's *Rockbound* acts as a gloss on Creighton's observations, for only the careys, "cursed birds of night," or the threat "o'dem haunts" can reduce the blond Viking, Gershom, to fear and trembling. He has inherited from Old Gershom a repertoire of stories, a healthy respect for haunts, and an ability to "present" a tale. In the ferocity of the storm on Barren Island, Gershom and David prepare for an evening of story-telling by boiling hot water for the rum, putting out lump sugar and lemon, and establishing the context of the narrative:

> "Dere's somethin' queer on dis island, too," said Gershom, "dough I don't understand rightly why, 'cause de Sanford folks tuk it away."
> "How's dat?" asked David, though he knew the story well.
> "You mind Johnny Publicover, de ghost catcher on Big Outpost?"
> "I minds him well, 'cause I lived nigh him when I was a gaffer."[48]

The tale is known to both men, as Debra Surette has pointed out in "Folklore in *Rockbound* and *John Paul's Rock,*" but they follow story-telling conventions, drawing comfort from the familiarity of the story and from the personal interaction the conventions provide". As the night progresses, the rum-drinking is part of the ritual, part of the measured presentation and anticipation of all the mysterious details. "The query and answer were made for no rhetorical effect," notes Day's speaker, "but for the purpose of allowing narrator and listener to pause long enough to take another draught of hot rum and hold it in the mouth a moment before letting the soul-kindling liquor trickle slowly down the gullet."[49] It is long past midnight when Gershom has completed his tale, having embellished it with his own touches of comedy, opinion, and detail. Day further enriches the presentation through

46 *Rockbound*, p. 72.

47 Helen Creighton, *Bluenose Ghosts* (Toronto, 1957), p. 280; quoted in Surette, "Folklore," p. 4.

48 *Rockbound*, pp. 108, 102, 115.

49 *Rockbound*, pp. 225-26; Surette, "Folklore," p. 8.

the vividness of Gershom's speech ("de ghos' fetches de back o' de schoolhouse whang, whang"), and through the dramatic irony of Gershom's confusing the "exorcising a ghost" with "exercising" one.[50] The result is an episode of humour, drama, and local colour that brings the central characters and their culture vividly alive. By turning to folktales like this, notes Surette, Day found an effective tool for creating a strong sense of place and for developing an "holistic approach to community."[51]

In spite of a number of requests in 1929-30 that *Rockbound* be reprinted,[52] the novel was not re-issued until 1973 when the University of Toronto Press published it with an introduction by Allan Bevan of the Dalhousie University English Department. In the years following original publication, Day brought out *John Paul's Rock* (1932) and *A Good Citizen* (1947). Crippling arthritis forced his early retirement as president of Union College in 1933, and in the succeeding years Day moved back to the Maritimes and enjoyed a sometime association with his *alma mater,* Mount Allison University. He also continued to write short stories and novels, turning at times to Mount Allison graduate, poet, and novelist Charles Bruce for advice on honing his fiction and submitting it to Canadian publishers. "I should like to send you my novel 'What Happened to Rosalie' that failed to win the Ryerson award, and get a criticism from you that might help me to amend it," he wrote Bruce from Lake Annis in May 1948; "...There is no one down here to whom I can turn for a worth-while criticism. I don't want *praise* or applesauce. Also can you tell me how to get hold of good literary agents in N.Y. Toronto and London. McLelland & Stuart [sic] are now reading my 'What The River Heard' which I wrote last year. It is very hard to judge one's own babies but both of these books seem to me to have some merit."[53]

In spite of the merits of these manuscripts, however, novels like "What the River Heard," "What Happened to Rosalie," and "Victory Garden" failed as sustained, fully unified narratives and were rejected by Scribner's, McClelland and Stewart, and a variety of other publishing houses Day approached. Often too crippled by arthritis at the end of his life to leave his bed, Day concluded a letter to Charles Bruce on Christmas Day 1949 with ruminations on the obscurity of contemporary literature and on the strengths of Bruce's own work in progress. "You have much talent," he noted, "and I

---

50 *Rockbound*, pp. 118-19, 117.

51 "Folklore," pp. 10, 38.

52 Day wrote on 18 May 1929 that he had no copies of *Rockbound* and hoped "some day that they will print another edition" (Day Papers, C240). In a letter to Day in 15 August 1930, Nella B. Henney of Doubleday, Doran & Company noted that the publisher had received a number of requests for *Rockbound* and *Autobiography of a Fisherman* but had no plans to republish the books. She offered to sell the plates for $100 a book.

53 Day to Bruce, 27 May 1948, Charles Bruce Papers, MS. 2.297.C38, DUA.

hope you'll have time to express more and more your nostalgia for our wind-
swept coast, and that when you come home you may be able to express the
joy of your return."[54] The note is both prophetic and revealing, coming as it
does just four years before the publication of Bruce's Nova Scotian novel *The
Channel Shore*, just seven months before Day's death on 30 July 1950,[55] and
some 30 years after the appearance of *Rockbound*, Day's own novel of the
"wind-swept coast."

54   Day to Bruce, 25 December 1949, *ibid.*

55   "Soldier, Author, Educator Passes Away on Sunday," *Yarmouth Light*, 3 August 1950; "Dr.
Frank Parker Day," *Union Alumnus*, Day Papers, M66.

The "Home Place" in
Modern Maritime Literature

My native community was, and mostly remains [writes Rick Rofihe in the *Dalhousie Magazine* in the winter of 1991], an area of small family farms, some villages and a few towns. There have been some changes in recent years since a large Europe-based manufacturing concern established itself in the area, operating 24 hours a day. As a regular wage does have its attractions over the vagaries of farming, agriculture there is gradually becoming a part-time affair — it's hard to keep milk cows when you're working the midnight-to-eight shift. There's an expression, "Goin' down home," which people in the county use to say that they're on their way to visit their childhood address, a place that's rarely more than 20 miles away....

I went down home one summer and was with my father when, looking to buy strawberries, he drove up a dirt road on a long, grassy slope to a farmhouse of some people he knew. The farmer, his wife and their son came out. I recognized her — she'd worked at a candy store that I'd frequented as a child. I recalled that she'd always taken time to talk to me, about the farm, her kids, their horses. Now, visiting years later, I was bracing myself to be asked where I was living these days. Somehow, grimy New York seemed especially inferior to this high country hill.

Her husband sent their son to get us some berries, apologizing that they didn't have too many this year, as things were busy what with the wife away in Paris, and only just getting back.

"Paris, France?" I asked her.

"Oh," she said, "Paris is wonderful — the company sent me over on a training trip. But it's nice to be home...and where's your home now?"

As she'd just come from a big city and had had a good time, I confidently blurted out, "New York City — right in Manhattan."

"New York." She gave me a big smile. "Oh, I loved New York. We were there in, gosh 1956...."[1]

This vignette does not abound with drama, but it does contain the threads of modern Maritime life. On the one hand there is the author of the piece, Rick Rofihe — teacher, children's writer, contributor to the *New Yorker* and the *New York Times* — who like generations before him has followed the well-trodden road of outmigration from the Maritime Provinces to seek a career

---

1   Rick Rofihe, "No place like home in the land that law forgot," *Dalhousie Magazine* (Winter 1991), p. 32.

elsewhere. On the other hand there is the farm couple — he still traditionally growing his strawberries "up a dirt road on a long grassy slope" on a "high country hill" and she, once a seller of candy, now a trainee for a European firm, newly back from Paris, newly integrated into the corporate world. The threads of the three Maritimes are here — the old, the new, the away — but all of them united and brought together by one thing — their common rootedness in a small South Shore Nova Scotian community — their common bond in being from "down home." "Down home," "the home place" — what writer, Clive Doucet of Grand Étang in Cape Breton calls "the village of my father and his father...a hometown of the mind and heart"[2] — makes a veiled appearance in Maritime Provinces literature in 1907 with the local colour writing of L.M. Montgomery's *Anne of Green Gables*, but for various reasons, gathers momentum in the 1920s. Why it begins to evolve in this period, and persists as a focus of such contemporary Maritime writers as David Adams Richards, George Elliott Clarke, Harry Bruce, Alistair MacLeod and Douglas Lochhead, is a subject for discussion. For surely, one may want to argue, "place" is a central image in any country's literature, and houses, buildings, villages dominate the imaginative landscape of much Canadian writing from Robertson Davies' Deptford and Margaret Laurence's Manawaka to Robert Kroetsch's "home place" on the prairie farm of "Seed Catalogue." But the emergence of the image in Maritime literature in the 1920s, it would seem, has its genesis in social, economic, and cultural realities on the east coast that distinguish it from similar images in other areas of Canada. For Davies and Laurence, Deptford and Manawaka play a role in the *bildungsroman* pattern of their novels. The towns are characterized by their parochialism, puritanism, and class divisiveness. Morag Gunn and Dunstan Ramsay spend major portions of their lives trying to free themselves from their towns' inhibiting influences and only late in life come to an acceptance of the fact that, as Dunstan puts it, "any new life must include Deptford. There was to be no release by muffling up the past."[3] In this sense, Morag and Dunstan are different from Robert Kroetsch's persona in "Seed Catalogue," who retrospectively sees in the "home place" the nurturing role of the mother in "planting" the speaker's poetic imagination against a prairie backdrop of shamanistic, male influences. In his poem, "The double hook:/ the home place"[4] is part of what Kroetsch has described elsewhere as the telling of our personal and national story: "In a sense we haven't got an identity until somebody tells our story. The fiction makes us real."[5] All of this is quite different from what occurs in Maritime Provinces literature where

---

2   Lesley Choyce, ed., *The Cape Breton Collection* (Porter's Lake, Nova Scotia, 1984), p. 55.

3   Robertson Davies, *Fifth Business* (New York, 1970), p. 121.

4   Robert Kroetsch, *Seed Catalogue* (Winnipeg, 1986), p. 21.

5   Robert Kroetsch, ed., *Creation* (Toronto, 1970), p. 63.

from the 1920s onward, the "home place" emerges as a symbol of cultural continuity and psychological identification in the face of social fragmentation, outmigration, and a continuing hardscrabble economy. Writers from Roger Viets in the eighteenth century to Charles G.D. Roberts in the twentieth had always drawn upon Maritime backgrounds to inform their works, but by the 1920s, the Maritime society that the Song Fishermen poets Andrew Merkel, Charles Bruce, Kenneth Leslie, and James D. Gillis faced was quite different from the Maritimes of the pre-war period. As historian E.R. Forbes has pointed out, the early 1920s saw the beginning of a long-term depression in the Maritime Provinces:

> Cut off from traditional markets by freight rates, with tariff protection undercut by inflation, rebates, and actual reductions, Maritime manufacturers were in a poor position to compete in a national economy. Already integrated into a branch-plant system controlled from central Canada, Maritime factories such as the Canada Car Company of Amherst or the Maritime Nail Company of Saint John were shut down, and the market served directly from central Canada. The British Empire Steel Corporation, which included a coal mining section with an output of five to seven million tons per year, was thrown into disarray. The corporation tried to pass losses on to its workers who, in turn, resisted with strikes every year from 1922 to 1925. By 1926 the large iron and steel section of the corporation was bankrupt and in the hands of a receiver. 42 per cent of the jobs in manufacturing disappeared in the region in the five years from 1920 to 1926. An estimated 15 to 20 per cent of the population left the region during the decade.[6]

The neglected houses that dotted the region in the years afterwards attested in human terms to the impact of the economic and social shifts taking place from the post 1920s years onwards. "The winter winds are bleak and drear," notes Cape Breton labour poet, Dawn Fraser, in 1925, "Methinks I better move from here."[7] Tables on the increase in population in Maritime counties such as Antigonish and Inverness in the 1921-1931 period reveal a -13.01 per cent and a -11.57 per cent decline respectively[8] and are typical of the pattern of outmigration across the region. As statistics, they reinforce the images emerging in Maritime literature in the interwar and post-World War II period

---

6   Ernest R. Forbes, *Aspects of Maritime Regionalism, 1867-1927* (Ottawa, 1983), p. 18.

7   Dawn Fraser, *Echoes From Labor's War* (Toronto, 1978). This is quoted in John G. Reid, *Six Crucial Decades* (Halifax, 1987), p. 170.

8   *The Maritime Provinces in Their Relation to the National Economy of Canada* (Ottawa, Dominion Bureau of Statistics, 1934), p. 10.

— the "fellows who keep the salt in the blood" as Charles Bruce notes in his poem "Words Are Never Enough" — who "give to the cities bordered with woods and grass/ A few homesick men, walking an alien street;/ A few women, remembering misty stars/ And the long grumbling sigh of the bay at night."[9] Consistent with the bittersweet images of exile developed here, Charles Bruce has frequently been one of the region's most representative literary figures in developing the image of the "home place." Physically removed himself from generations of rootedness on the Guysborough or "Channel Shore" of his novel of that name, Bruce articulated in that 1954 work a vision of the "home place" as almost a moral force informing the wider world. A centre of psychological identification for those who left it, "it was not a little world, now, from which people went and to which they sometimes returned, but a living part of a larger world, a part of the whole thing, like Halifax or Boston or Montreal. He saw the Shore now not as the one place loved and friendly and known, but as his own particular part of something larger, embracing all, the bright and the ugly, the familiar and the strange."[10]

This image of the "home place" as the nurturer not only of local tradition but also of a wider social universe runs counter to current critical charges by cultural historian Ian McKay that much Maritime literature is merely a literature of nostalgia created by middle class writers who idealize a pastoral, golden age as part of "a culture of consolation." Lacking viable political and economic alternatives to outmigration and financial decline in the interwar period, argues McKay, middle class intellectuals and artists in the region often tended to turn a negative stereotype of the Maritimes into a positive one, re-imagining "Communities lacking modern amenities and precariously dependent upon natural resources...as unspoiled hamlets, havens of authenticity in an artificial world." From tourism to literature is a very small step in McKay's thesis. If you can no longer march with the band of progress, then it may be comforting to fall back on a memory of a golden age — a "home place," if you will, of "loving" and "friendliness" and "knowing." From the invention of Peggy's Cove as an icon of regional identity, notes McKay, "the transition could as aptly be traced in regional literature, in the mass enthusiasm for the schooner *Bluenose*, and in the conscious reinvention and manipulation of Scottish traditions."[11]

McKay's thesis offers a tempting way of approaching the image of the "home place" in modern Maritime literature, since it is, to an extent, pastoral

---

9   Charles Bruce, *The Mulgrave Road. Selected Poems of Charles Bruce* (Porter's Lake, Nova Scotia, 1984), p. 52.

10 Charles Bruce, *The Channel Shore* (Toronto, 1957), p. 261.

11 Ian McKay, "Among the Fisherfolk: J.F.B. Livesay and the Invention of Peggy's Cove", *Journal of Canadian Studies*, 23, 1 & 2 (Spring/ Summer 1988), pp. 23-45.

or nostalgic in tone. But to dismiss this literature as static, merely the product of middle class romanticization, is to ignore the elements of realism, irony, and economic cynicism permeating much of it. Bruce may celebrate in "Words Are Never Enough" the quiet moment at work's end when the men sit in the sun in idle talk, but there is no mitigating the "crooked fingers," "aching thighs," and "trenchant bite/Of cold salt water"[12] that make their lives physically and financially precarious. "The real-down-homer is a realist," notes Bruce in "That's why we Maritimers head home": "He (or his father) came from a place where hard work was and is done. He remembers the look of the bay at sunrise on a July morning before the wind makes up, and the smell of wild roses. He also remembers the feel of snow down the back of his neck, the way a shoulder aches from a crosscut saw, and the weight of a barrel of herring on a handbarrow."[13] Nor is the lyricism of Ernest Buckler's *Ox Bells and Fireflies* unmarked by a vision of death, decay, and irony: "the mouse blood on the frozen crust. The bag of day-old kittens in the pail drowned with their eyes shut. The leak in the hen pen" sliming "the droppings on the sodden straw. And old men with a milky film over their pupils" tapping "their way querulously with their canes to the outhouse."[14] Reinforcing these realistic elements (a realism that caused Ironbounders to object in 1928 to the portrayal of themselves in Frank Parker Day's novel *Rockbound*) is a texture of language, domestic imagery, and detail convincing in its depiction of lived life. "I've just read my leisurely way through *Ox Bells and Fireflies*," Charles Bruce was to write Buckler in 1969,

> and this note is just to say that I have enjoyed greatly meeting again the kind of people I grew up among, and hearing some of the expressions — "chipyard," "shop," and "getting a chance" from place to place — that were part of their speech and mine.
>
> Part of the whatever-it-is of Nova Scotia is the difference a man runs into, geographical and racial, between places within a few miles of each other. Eastern Guysborough County, where I grew up, is rather different from The Valley (as we always called your part of the world); even in our own little bailiwick we on the north shore of Chedabucto Bay, mostly English, Scots and Irish, were somewhat different from the descendants of Hessians five or six miles away across the bay. In even narrower terms, we who lived west of St. Francis Harbor were somewhat different from the Irish Catholic down-alongers who lived at St. Francis and from there along to Sand Point (They were given to card-laying, dancing etc., which were not tolerated around Port

---

12 Bruce, *The Mulgrave Road*, pp. 49-50.

13 Charles Bruce, "That's why we Maritimers head home," *Mayfair* (July 1955), p. 20.

14 Ernest Buckler, *Ox Bells and Fireflies* (Toronto, 1974), p. 302.

Shoreham and Manchester). But beneath the difference runs some kind of common tide." [15]

This kind of cultural shading conveyed as convincingly and as detailedly in Bruce's fiction and poetry as in his correspondence, finds echo in other literary depictions of the "home place" ranging from David Adams Richards' stylized Miramichi of the 1970s and 1980s to George Elliot Clarke's Whylah Falls of 1990. Language and idiom, key signatures of folk culture, speak of a zest in verbal tradition and invention, not stasis. "Down home the small boy never throws a stone," notes Bruce. "He does not chase an enemy. He takes after him. And when he's overhauled him he does not punch him in the nose. He knocks him into the middle of next week."[16] "People in rural and Maritime areas both have inherited and are proud of a certain tradition of speaking which is relatively fixed," argues Professor Lewis J. Poteet, who has done much research on the speech of the South Shore of Nova Scotia, "and from that tradition I believe they inherit a taste for making new words and phrases colourful in the same way as those learned from their grand-parents."[17] Or, as George Elliott Clarke notes of Black vernacular, "It's a form of speaking the self, identifying the self, and it has a right to be set free."[18] The literary language of the "home place" repeatedly illustrates Poteet and Clarke's claim, whether in the form of David Richards' stylized Miramichi "ya" in *The Coming of Winter* ["Ya and seven bucks is a bit of a burn"; "Oh hell I know her, ya"][19] or in the cast of the Lunenburg dialect of Frank Parker Day's *Rockbound* ["Why, dat ghost...were dat audacious he used to whang on de back o'de church at evening meetin"]. In *Whylah Falls* (1990), his collection of poems celebrating a symbolic Black community where the British Crown settled coloured Loyalists after the American Revolution, George Elliott Clarke surprises expectations by sensuously employing the language of regional food — rappie pie, steamed fiddleheads, gaspereau boiled in vinegar — as part of his textural self-identification:

> Her Jarvis County cuisine, gumboing the salty recipes of Fundy
> Acadians, the starchy diets of South Shore Loyalists, and the fishy

---

15   Charles Bruce to Ernest Buckler, Charles Bruce Papers, Dal. Ms. 2, 297, Dalhousie University Archives.

16   Bruce, "That's why we Maritimers head home," p. 63.

17   Quoted in Mavor Moore, "Insight Gleaned from the Mail," *Globe and Mail* (26 October 1985).

18   Dan Bortolotti, "The Vernacular Music of George Elliott Clarke," *Books In Canada*, Vol. XX, No. 7 (October 1991), p. 20.

19   David Adams Richards, *The Coming of Winter* (Ottawa, 1974), pp. 32 and 34; Frank Parker Day, *Rockbound* (Toronto, 1989 [1928]), p. 115.

tastes of Coloured Refugees, includes rappie pie, sweet potato pie, pollen pancakes, steamed fiddleheads, baked cabbage, fried clams, dandelion beer, gaspereau boiled in vinegar, and basic black-and-blue berries. For breakfast, Cora offers fried eggs, sausages, orange marmalade, and toast, washed down with rich coffee. Her tastes are eccentric, exotic, eclectic. Her carrot cake consists of whole carrots whose green, leafy tops sprout from brown, earthen icing, and whose orange roots taper all the way to the cake's floor. She bakes apple tree leaves, blossoms, seeds, and bark into her apple pies. Cora is the concrete poet of food.[20]

There is something fluid and ongoing and alive in this application of "gumboing" culinary language to domestic rituals that transcends centuries and imaginatively unites the eighteenth-century origins of Clarke's "home place" to his twentieth-century exploration of it. Place: inherited customs: work rhythms: exile: return — all merge in Clarke's poem sequence as a celebration of a life force that carries the "home place" beyond the image of sentimentality and stasis into something more organic and breathing and changing. "Sunshine illumines the mirage of literature," Clarke writes, "how everyone uses words to create a truth he or she can trust and live within."[21] Or, to recall Robert Kroetsch, it is the "telling" of the story that helps to "make us real." The telling may make us real, but words, as Charles Bruce tells us in his poem "are never enough." For the writer of literature, articulating the nature of Maritime identity is a nebulous and elusive process. Being a Maritimer is something felt in the blood and in the bone. It is knowing, as fiction writer Alistair MacLeod puts it in the title of his first book, the "salt" in "your blood." This is the romanticism that could substantiate Ian McKay's remarks, but there is nothing forced about a sense of tradition — nothing "invented" — when in MacLeod's "The Closing Down of Summer," the Cape Breton miners travel world wide in search of their profession but carry with them always sprigs of Island spruce:

> ...and take them with us to Africa as mementos or talismans or symbols of identity. Much as our Highland ancestors, for centuries, fashioned crude badges of heather or of whortle-berries to accompany them on the battlefields of the world. Perhaps so that in the closeness of their work with death they might find nearness to their homes and an intensified realization of themselves. [22]

---

20   George Elliott Clarke, *Whylah Falls* (Winlaw, British Columbia, 1990), p. 36.

21   *Ibid.*, p. 13.

22   Alistair MacLeod, *As Birds Bring Forth The Sun* (Toronto, 1986), p. 16. When a version of this paper was presented at the British Association for Canadian Studies conference at

An "intensified realization" of *self* is what the "home place" conveys in Maritime literature. Born in the catalyst of 1920s financial and social fragmentation, it has continued throughout the outmigration and declining economic and political influence of the post-1920s years to illuminate Maritime literature with a sense of cultural continuity and psychological identification. "In clamour of great cities," writes Sophie Almon Hensley, "I could see,/ Eyes closed, the marshes that I loved, the stream/ Of plover, hear the raucous call of crows." Always "alien, nationless," when away "from St. Mary's Bay/ From little sleepy towns of Gaspereaux," she returns in old age, "in the gloam/ My eventide" to "home."[23] In doing so, she speaks for generations of Maritime writers and readers who physically and imaginatively see in the "home place" the essence of their Maritime identity.

Nottingham, England, in April 1991, Professor Andrew Wainwright of Dalhousie University pointed out that much of the writing about the "home place" has been done retrospectively by writers like Bruce, Buckler, Hensley, MacLeod, Clarke, etc., who have become educated and have left the region. This is an extremely interesting point and one that I have not developed in the paper. Some writers, like David Adams Richards, have, however, not left the region. In the case of Bruce, Hensley, Buckler, and Lochhead, they later returned to the region. Alistair MacLeod continues to maintain his contact during summers and sabbaticals. However, the whole question of how the expatriate stance affects writing about the "home place," (as raised by Professor Wainwright) needs to be explored.

23   Sophia M. Hensley, "Repatriated," *Dalhousie Review*, 13, No. 4 (January, 1934), p. 439. I am grateful to Dr. Carole Gerson, Simon Fraser University, for calling my attention to this poem.

INDEX